AIDS: PSYCHIATRIC AND PSYCHOSOCIAL PERSPECTIVES

AIDS:

PSYCHIATRIC AND PSYCHOSOCIAL PERSPECTIVES

Edited by
LESLIE PAINE

CHAPMAN AND HALL

LONDON • NEW YORK • TOKYO • MELBOURNE • MADRAS

UK	Chapman and Hall, 2–6 Boundary Row, London SE1 8HN
USA	Chapman and Hall, 29 West 35th Street, New York NY 10001
JAPAN	Chapman and Hall Japan, Thomson Publishing Japan, Hirakawacho Nemoto Building, 7F, 1-7-11 Hirakawa-cho, Chiyoda-ku, Tokyo 102
AUSTRALIA	Chapman and Hall Australia, Thomas Nelson Australia, 480 La Trobe Street, PO Box 4725, Melbourne 3000
INDIA	Chapman and Hall India, R. Seshadri, 32 Second Main Road, CIT East, Madras 600 035

First edition 1988
Reprinted 1990

© 1988 Leslie Paine

Printed and bound in Great Britain by
Biddles Ltd, Guildford and King's Lynn

ISBN 0 412 38340 3

British Library Cataloguing in Publication Data

AIDS : psychiatric and psychosocial
  perspectives.
  1. AIDS – Psychological aspects
  2. AIDS – Social aspects
  I. Paine, Leslie
  616.9′792′0019   RC607.A26
  ISBN 0 412 38340 3

Library of Congress Cataloging in Publication Data

AIDS, psychiatric and psychosocial perspectives/edited by Leslie
  Paine.
    p. cm.
  Based on a conference held at the Institute of Psychiatry on Feb.
  27, 1987, sponsored jointly by Association of Directors of Social
  Services and others.
  Includes index.
  ISBN (invalid) 0 412 38340 3
  1. AIDS (Disease) – Psychological aspects – Congresses. 2. AIDS
  (Disease) – Social aspects – Congresses.   3. AIDS (Disease) – Patients –
  Mental health – Congresses.   I. Paine, Leslie.   II. Association of
  Directors of Social Services (Great Britain)
    [DNLM: 1. Acquired Immunodeficiency Syndrome – psychology –
  congresses.   WD308   A288392]
  RC607.A26A34885   1988
  616.9′792′0019 – dc 19
  DNLM/DLC
  for Library of Congress   87-30512

Contents

Contributors

Professor R.H. Cawley, Department of Psychological Medicine, Institute of Psychiatry and King's College School of Medicine and Dentistry, London.

Dr James W. Dilley, Director, AIDS Health Project, University of California, San Francisco.

Professor A.M. Geddes, Department of Medicine, University of Birmingham.

Dr John Green, District Clinical Psychologist, St Mary's Hospital, London.

Riva Miller, AIDS Counselling Co-ordinator, Hampstead Health Authority, London.

Denise Platt, Director of Social Services, Hammersmith and Fulham, London.

Dr J.L. Reed, Senior Principal Medical Officer, Mental Health Division, Department of Health and Social Security, London.

Dr J. Roy Robertson, General Practitioner, Edinburgh Drug Addiction Study.

Ben Thomas, Tutor, School of Nursing, Bethlem Royal and Maudsley Hospitals, London.

Dr Jonathan Weber, Chester Beatty Laboratories, Institute of Cancer Research, London.

Introduction

R.H. Cawley

During the brief years since its appearance, the AIDS virus
(human immunodeficiency virus, HIV) has secured its place as
one of the significant and sinister medical puzzles of this or any
other generation. It has also achieved eminence as providing
some of the most compelling examples of interaction between
biomedical and psychosocial variables.

AIDS is a disease caused by a germ, yet none of the well-tried
procedures of immunisation or treatment by chemicals or
antibiotics can, in the foreseeable future, have any effect beyond
the palliative. This is because of the novel set of biological
mechanisms, scientifically as challenging as they are awesome,
whereby the virus invades and takes over the cells which
comprise the body's major defence system.

As there is no cure and no preventive treatment, the disease
can be avoided only by making sure the organism doesn't enter
the body.

It is just as well that, even though the disease is endemic, the
organism isn't everywhere. Indeed it cannot exist in more than
a few places. It is not very infectious and can't survive outside
the human body. Even when there is close contact with those
most severely affected, the virus can invade the body only
through sexual activity or by being introduced into the blood
stream.

Now that certain lessons have been learned, some of the

tragedies will not recur, for laboratory procedures can virtually guarantee the purity of substances — including blood itself — used for intravenous infusion in treating people with haemophilia. All else now depends on human behaviour — sexual activity, especially but not exclusively involving homosexual men, and the behaviour of people dependent upon opiates and other substances self-administered intravenously.

So in the present state of our knowledge the absolute determinants of the spread of AIDS are personal, behavioural and social, saturated with human emotions, motivations and values.

(AIDS and related conditions occur mostly in young people.) They are progressive, distressing and debilitating illnesses, ultimately fatal. Both acute and chronic brain affections — causing mental confusion and dementia — may accompany HIV infection, either as a result of the organism itself invading cells in the brain, or as complications of the opportunistic infections which are the hallmark of full-blown AIDS.

In addition it is hardly surprising that a wide range of adverse emotional reactions are regularly reported in HIV-positive people. The illness is devastating and destructive of life; the individual's reactions are likely to be the more painful and severe because the disease is spread by sexual encounters and by the sharing of needles by those who abuse drugs. Because of the nature of the disease itself therefore, an elaborate framework of emotional and practical support and care in the community is called for. This is a heavy task for the statutory and voluntary social agencies.

Besides people who have become ill, those who are infected (HIV-positive) and remain well have their own predicaments for which they need help and support. In addition many who are not ill and not carriers are greatly influenced by the presence of the AIDS virus in the community. The partners of those affected, families and other carers carry heavy emotional burdens. So do people who consider themselves at risk — with or without reason. AIDS-related anxiety may lead to distressing phobic and hypochondriacal states in otherwise healthy people.

Indeed it seems that every manifestation of the virus, direct and indirect, provides a set of problems for multidisciplinary psychosocial and medical care. An extraordinarily wide range of

professions, charitable organisations and volunteers are impli-
cated. The needs are resounding and the opportunities are great:
there is more than enough room for everybody to contribute.
Failures of understanding, collaboration or harmonisation of
effort would be tragic.

In early 1986 the DHSS Expert Advisory Group on AIDS
appointed a sub-group with the brief to explore the psychiatric
and psychosocial aspects of AIDS. The multidisciplinary
conference on this topic, held at the Institute of Psychiatry on 27
February 1987, was one result. Some 220 people, from a wide
variety of professional and other caring groups, attended. As
space was limited, about 100 had their applications returned. In
planning the meeting it was recognised that the frameworks
necessary for comprehending the psychological and social
aspects could be built only on the solid ground of what is at
present known about the biology of the virus and the medical
consequences of infection.

This publication is a product of the conference. It is a position
paper setting out what appear at this stage to be the outstanding
psychiatric and psychosocial dimensions of AIDS and related
disorders, and exploring possible directions for consolidating
and further developing the understanding necessary for
appropriate service developments.

It deliberately falls short of presenting a firm list of conclu-
sions and recommendations. The task of the conference was to
explore a wide range of themes: any attempt at conclusion and
closure could only have been presumptuous and signified failure.

In the matter of comprehending the psychosocial implications
of the AIDS virus and laying down the required courses of
action, we have barely reached the end of the beginning.

Acknowledgements

The conference was sponsored jointly by

Association of Directors of Social Services
AVERT (AIDS Virus Education and Research Trust)
British Association of Social Workers
British Psychological Society
Department of Health & Social Security
Institute of Psychiatry
King's College School of Medicine and Dentistry
Royal College of Nursing
Royal College of Psychiatrists
SCODA
Terrence Higgins Trust

The editor is pleased to acknowledge a grant from AVERT which has enabled this book to be prepared for publication.

1

The Biology of HIV

Jonathan Weber

AIDS and the AIDS-associated syndromes are new phenomena first recognised only six years ago, in the spring of 1981, and seen only retrospectively in the western world back to 1979. The sudden appearance of this syndrome led to considerable confusion in the medical profession as to possible aetiology. Fortunately, our knowledge and understanding of AIDS changed dramatically between 1983 and 1984. In the May of 1983, Françoise Barre-Sinoussi, working in Dr Montagnier's laboratory at the Institut Pasteur in Paris, isolated a novel retrovirus from cells of a patient with persistent generalised lymphadenopathy (PGL), which we now recognise as being one of the clinical conditions caused by the AIDS virus.

That virus, LAV-1, as shown in the electron micrograph (Figure 1.1) has a fragile outer envelope containing lipid, which is relatively easily disrupted, surrounding a condensed core of very characteristic shape, which contains the viral RNA, surrounded by the core proteins.

The virus grows predominately in T-lymphocytes and can be grown *in vitro* in tissue culture, where it results in a lytic infection, killing the lymphocytes in which it grows. If infected T4$^+$ lymphocytes are stimulated and made to divide, for example by using a mitogen, the virus is encouraged to replicate. Mature viral particles can then be observed 'budding' from the surface of infected cells. These particles are infectious and can infect

Figure 1.1: Electron micrograph of the LAV-1 virus

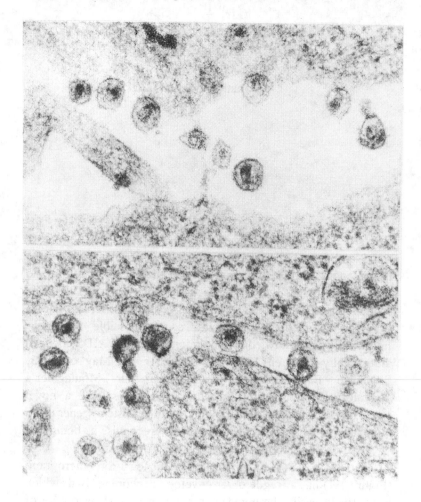

other cells. As most infected cells are lysed by the AIDS virus, establishing a persistent infection was initially difficult.

This is a virus which replicates and divides in activated lymphocytes. When it is integrated within the genetic materials of host cells it may be completely inactive and latent, but on activation of the cell there is a sudden liberation of new viral particles into the extracellular fluid bathing that cell.

The virus lives by and large within cells of the immune system within the peripheral blood. When these cells divide, viral particles are given off into the plasma, and therefore into all the plasma-derived bodily fluids, such as saliva, tears and, more importantly, seminal fluid, and fluid in the vagina and cervix. All of these bodily fluids, and all the body's extracellular fluids, may contain viral particles in low concentration. However, as discussed below, the presence of viral particles is not directly related to infectivity.

These are the viral mechanisms which explain the epidemiological pattern of the disease. The presence of viral particles in blood and semen leads to infection in recipients by inoculation.

The nomenclature of the AIDS virus is still in confusion, despite efforts at simplification. The first virus isolated in 1983 was called LAV-1. Subsequently, a similar virus was isolated in the United States by Robert Gallo, and he termed this HTLV-III. HTLV-III was grown initially in peripheral blood lymphocytes, where it produced the same lytic infection as LAV-1, making a permanently producing cell line impossible. Eventually, in early 1984, Mikolas Popovic in Dr Gallo's laboratory succeeded in permanently infecting a cell line called H9. This enabled the virus to be produced in large quantities, and led to the development of assays which definitively and causally associated this new retrovirus with the disease of AIDS. Because of confusion over nomenclature, renaming has taken place, and the AIDS virus, which is the sole cause of AIDS and associated conditions, is now referred to internationally as a lentivirus, called the human immunodeficiency virus type 1 (HIV-1).

This virus — HIV-1 — is now pandemic throughout the world, being reported from over 109 countries. Indeed any country which has an airport runway long enough to take a

Boeing 747 will be likely to have HIV present in the population. Many countries, including all of Western Europe, now have endemic transmission of HIV; this means that transmission of HIV is a self-sustaining epidemic in the UK, not relying on infection acquired abroad.

Within the past year, however, a new focus of AIDS has emerged in West Africa in which a different virus is causing the same disease. The differences between the viruses are relatively small, and this new West African virus is called either HIV-2, LAV-2 or HTLV-IV — an unnecessary confusion which may be resolved by general agreement to use the description HIV-2.

Essentially these viruses are different virologically, particularly in the envelope region, but the same biologically. They cause the same disease in the body, and they have exactly the same distribution in terms of sexual dissemination and the development of AIDS in infected patients. In addition, both HIV-1 and HIV-2 share identical cell tropisms for the T4 antigen.

This second new isolate, HIV-2, has emerged chiefly in West African countries such as Senegal, Guinea–Bissau and Ivory Coast. We are still largely unaware of the mechanism underlying the emergence of HIV-1 or HIV-2 as new pathogens of man, and we have a very limited understanding both of its natural evolution and its relationship to the simian immunodeficiency viruses (SIV) which have been shown to occur in old world monkeys. These SIVs are lentiviruses with close similarity to HIV, and have been found in particular in African monkeys such as vervets, the African green monkey and also certain mangabeys and other diverse species of old world monkeys. The SIVs or simian immunodeficiency viruses are the likeliest origin for the human viruses which cause AIDS, but the actual details of possible modes of transmission between a simian reservoir and a human epidemic are still unclear. The similar tropism for all the simian SIV viruses, and the HIV-1 and HIV-2 for the T4 molecular, points to a conserved evolutionary history.

These HIV and SIV viruses are all retroviruses, which means that they are RNA viruses whose genetic material consists of RNA, but which have a unique enzyme called reverse transcriptase which enables them to make a DNA copy of themselves. The central dogma propounded by Watson and Crick in molecular

Figure 1.2: 'Knobs' on outer coat of AIDS virus (see text)

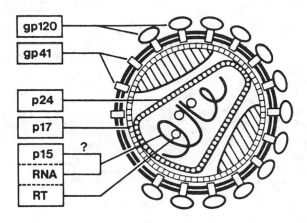

biology is that DNA is the repository of genetic information which produced RNA, which in turn produced proteins, of which living matter is constituted. It was seen as a one-way process. Retroviruses are the only known organisms in which a DNA copy is made of an RNA template and, because they can develop a DNA copy of themselves, this can integrate into our own genetic material. In this respect they are not completely different from many DNA viruses — such as herpes viruses — since they also can integrate into our genetic material.

Once we are infected by any of these retroviruses or DNA viruses we are infected for life, or certainly for the life of the cell, because once integrated, the viral genome cannot be eradicated. However, it is very likely that damage is only done when the integrated genome has actually been replicated and viral proteins are being expressed on the cell surface.

The AIDS virus itself has an outer coat with a series of knobs on it, and these knobs are critical (Figure 1.2). The interaction between the target cell and the virus takes place exclusively through recognition of these knobs, which are the principal envelope protein, gp120. This envelope protein is anchored to the virus by a trans-membrane protein — gp 41; and inside the virus is a central core, with the coil of RNA within it, and the

5

Figure 1.3: The HIV cell cycle

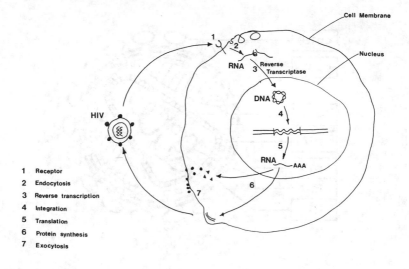

1   Receptor
2   Endocytosis
3   Reverse transcription
4   Integration
5   Translation
6   Protein synthesis
7   Exocytosis

unique retroviral enzyme — the reverse transcriptase which enables it to make its own DNA copy.

The life cycle of these retroviruses is extremely straight-forward (Figure 1.3). Free viral particles have to enter a suscep-tible cell, and by so doing must bind to a specific receptor on the cell surface. We know that this receptor is a particular molecule on the surface which we call CD4 (T4). This was recognised initially as a molecule on certain immunologically active cells such as $T4^+$ lymphocytes (helper T-lymphocytes); it is likely that CD4 is the 'recognition' signal by which cells of the immune system recognise one another and interact. The CD4 molecule appears to be the specific receptor for all the HIV and SIV viruses.

It is because we know the distribution of the receptor (CD4 molecule) that we also know exactly which cells can be infected *in vivo*, because if cells lack this receptor on their cell surface then they cannot be infected. After the virus is bound to the receptor it has to enter the cell — probably via active endocytosis — and replication occurs through the reverse transcriptase enzyme, a DNA copy being formed which then integrates into our own genetic material (Figure 1.3). Once integrated, it stays integrated, and if the viral DNA is latent, it will not damage the cell. But when the virus replicates, in other words, when messenger RNA is produced from this integrated DNA and virus proteins are produced, these, for reasons about which we cannot be certain, appear to be toxic to the cell and cause premature senility in those that are infected. Such cells die early, and it is the loss of these cells that leads to the disease we know as AIDS, and other related phenomena. The virus then buds off from the surface of the cells, and free viral particles are formed which can go off and infect other cells distantly.

As already mentioned, not all cells in the body contain this CD4 molecule on the cell surface. We know that it is present on 60 per cent of T lymphocytes, particularly a sub-set of T lymphocytes called the helper or inducer sub-set. These cells are clearly present in peripheral blood and to a lesser extent in lymph nodes, but they are really present throughout the body.

About 60 per cent of the lymphocytes in our body are CD4$^+$ lymphocytes, and these are all infectable. They are the commonest cells to be infected in the body by the AIDS virus, and it is the loss of these cells which leads principally to causation of the disease recognised as AIDS, i.e. the direct loss of the cellular immune system after HIV infection that leads to the development of disease. These helper lymphocytes are responsible for the first recognition of foreign antigens, and T-helper destruction paralyses the cellular immune system.

We also know that some B lymphocytes — i.e. antibody-producing lymphocytes — may also be infected, and that another group of immunologically active cells, called monocytes or macrophages, may also carry the CD4 molecule on their cell surface and therefore also be infected by HIV. The relevance of HIV infection in these sites is currently unknown.

These cells have a much wider distribution because macrophages are widely dispersed in tissues, and certainly they can be present deep in the skin, as Langerhans cells, and in the lung. Alveolar macrophages are infectable by this virus, and certainly much of the clinical pattern that we see may be due to a combination of loss of T lymphocytes, to infection of macrophages at specific sites, and to loss of action of local macrophages and other immunologically active cells.

Most importantly there exists a group of cells, in the central nervous system, called microglial cells. All cells in the central nervous system are either neurons or glia. Neurons are the nerve cells themselves. Glia are the supporting cells for neurons, and include astrocytes, oligodendrocytes (which are the central nervous system equivalent of Schwann cells) and microglia. By their name, microglia might seem to be derived from cells of the central nervous system. In fact they are not; microglia are probably bone-marrow-derived macrophages which, because they are like any other macrophages in the body, can be infected by HIV.

If, for example, we look at patients who have died of the AIDS-related dementia, which will be described in detail elsewhere, many of the microglia in the CNS are infected by HIV. A careful survey of cells in the CNS at post-mortem of HIV-infected patients reveals that *all* the infected cells appear to be of macrophage or lymphocyte origin. However, a small proportion of the infected cells may have the characteristics of a glial cell known as an oligodendrocyte.

Although the neurons are not infected *in vivo*, *in vitro* experiments show a wider range of astrocytes and other glial cells are infectable by HIV. However, the infection is not productive, and the HIV genome only latently integrates into the glia. The glial cells are not destroyed by HIV. Pathogenesis of HIV disease following infection is still unclear. However, there are three ways in which HIV causes disease *in vivo*:

(1) primary HIV effect — lytic action on infected cells;

(2) secondary opportunist infections — e.g. CNS toxoplasmosis;

(3) opportunist tumours — e.g. CNS B cell lymphoma

The primary HIV disease is that caused directly by the lytic action of HIV, as described above. The destruction of infected $T4^+$ cells leading to cellular immunosuppression and the destruction of cells in the CNS leading to dementia are primary effects. It is possible that there are also primary effects on the gut.

Secondary opportunist infections arise when the cellular

immune system has been paralysed by HIV infection and destruction of T4$^+$ cells. Many bacterial infections are resisted and controlled by our humoral (antibody) mediated immunity. Other infections, particularly protozoal, viral and fungal infections, are controlled more by cellular immunity. One example is *Pneumocystis carinii*. This protozoal organism probably infects us all in childhood, causing no disease, but leaving latent cysts in our lungs. When our cellular immune system is intact, immune surveillance results in total repression of *Pneumocystis*. However, when the cellular immunity is paralysed by the HIV virus then this *Pneumocystis carinii* organism can proliferate and cause active pneumonia. So these opportunist infections are by and large endogenous infections, infections we have had on board for a long time but which normally do not cause disease.

Then there are the opportunist tumours, such as Kaposi's sarcoma (KS). An opportunist tumour, one assumes, must almost invariably be caused by another virus. One of the tumours we see is the lymphoma caused by a herpes virus, called Epstein Barr virus, which, in the context of loss of immune surveillance, proliferates in these virally infected cells and leads to the development of a B-cell (Burkitt-type) lymphoma. Kaposi's sarcoma must also be caused by a virus, but this has not yet been discovered.

These therefore are the only ways whereby the AIDS virus causes disease within the CNS: disease caused by direct, lytic, HIV infection of CNS glial cells and microglia; opportunist infections with cerebral toxoplasmosis or cryptococcal meningitis; and opportunist tumours such as CNS B-cell lymphoma. Kaposi's sarcoma, though commonly found in AIDS patients, is rarely seen in the CNS.

We know that the HIV virus is present in the CNS because of three key pieces of work. Firstly, George Shaw from Dr Gallo's laboratory at NIH showed by a DNA hybridisation technique that actual HIV virus is present within the brains of AIDS patients with dementia. Secondly, David Ho in Boston demonstrated that he can culture the HIV virus from cerebrospinal fluids taken from patients with AIDS. And thirdly, Martin, also from Washington, showed that virtually all the cells within the central nervous system, which were infected by the virus, were in fact macrophage cells, which were also T4$^+$. These three experiments show circumstantially (though strongly) that HIV is directly involved in CNS disease in AIDS.

When we infect susceptible T4$^+$ cells in culture with the AIDS virus they come together and fuse, to produce giant cells or syncytial formations. These multinucleate clumps of cells then die, and this is one of the mechanisms by which the disease is possibly caused. This has not been demonstrated as occurring within HIV-infected CNS cells, yet remains a possible route for the pathogenesis of HIV in the CNS. Other methods of pathogenicity in the CNS remain open. It is conceivable that a cell-mediated attack on virally infected cells causes the AIDS-related dementia; more research is required. Similarly, the role of non-productive latent infection of CNS glial cells needs to be elucidated.

There is no treatment at the moment for this disease. However, because the HIV life cycle contains steps such as reverse transcription (RT) which is uniquely retroviral, it is possible to look at anti-viral drugs. One RT inhibitor, developed by the Wellcome Foundation, called azidothymidine (AZT, Retrovir, Zovidarine) has now been licensed for use in the UK. This drug terminates the transcription of proviral DNA from the viral RNA templates by terminating the growing DNA chain, therefore inhibiting viral replication. AZT has been demonstrated to prolong the life of patients with AIDS, but is not curative. There is a significant toxicity of AZT against bone marrow red blood cell precursors, and it is unlikely that AZT will benefit asymptomatic carriers of HIV, because of the hazards of bone marrow toxicity.

A recent report suggests that two out of four patients with AIDS-related dementia responded to AZT therapy, but this observation requires considerable confirmation. Similarly there is no vaccine available for AIDS and unfortunately none at present is in the pipeline. I and other scientists, however, remain optimistic that one may be discovered in the future.

Meanwhile, however, the only way of controlling the epidemic spread of the disease is through health education and counselling. I cannot stress too strongly that in consequence, while the scientific account I have just presented here is fascinating intellectually, it is what happens in practice with the counselling of infected people that is really critical for us all at this moment.

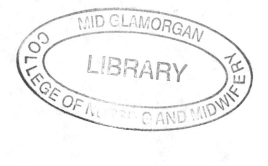

2

Epidemiology, Control of Infection, Medical Treatments

A.M. Geddes

Historians will remember that the great plagues of the Middle Ages were highly infectious and carried a large mortality: the Black Death, for example, halved the population of this country. There is a tendency, particularly in the popular press, when discussing the epidemiology of AIDS, to compare it with such plagues. Such a comparison is misconceived — AIDS is not a highly infectious disease.

Dr Jonathan Weber has already indicated in the previous chapter, that almost certainly the acquired immune deficiency syndrome is new. Other infections which are referred to as new, such as Legionnaire's disease, or Lassa fever, are almost certainly not. They have just been recognised recently, as a result of improved laboratory techniques. But there is very good epidemiological evidence that AIDS is new.

Where did it come from? Probably from Central Africa, although the final link with primates in Central Africa has not definitively been made. What is true, however is that there is a vast epidemic of AIDS in Africa, particularly in Central Africa, and this epidemic is spreading up East Africa, Uganda and Nigeria, and also now appearing in West Africa.

In Africa, AIDS appears to be a heterosexually transmitted disease, a situation that is the opposite of that which exists in the temperate climates where, as is well known, the homosexual is the principal victim, at least at the present time.

Table 2.1: AIDS, United States, December 1986 (total = 28,098)

	Male	Female	Paediatric
Homosexual/bisexual	18,162	—	
Intravenous drug abuser	3760	963	
Homosexual/intravenous drug abuser	2165	—	
Haemophilia/bleeding disorder	233	7	
Heterosexual contact			
United States	81	404	
Other country	461	110	
Transfusion acquired	324	181	
No information	648	205	
Totals	25,834	1870	394

And while we are considering Africa in the context, a question that is often asked is — can HIV infection be transmitted by mosquitoes, or by tsetse flies? There is now fairly firm evidence that tsetse flies and mosquitoes do not transmit HIV. Professor Arie Zuckerman at the London School of Hygiene and Tropical Medicine has tried to infect several different species of mosquito with this virus and has been unsuccessful. Another good reason for suggesting that it is not transmitted by mosquitoes is that in Africa it is a disease of the sexually active and not of children. If it were transmitted by mosquitoes we would see the disease in children.

How did the infection get from Africa to Europe?

It seems most likely that it started to break out of Africa when labourers from the Caribbean island of Haiti went to work in Zaire, contracted the infection heterosexually, and took it back home to a country which, by great misfortune, happened to be the playground of the promiscuous North American homosexual man. In that way it got back to North America and then across the Atlantic to Europe.

A little later a second prong attack was heterosexually transmitted directly northwards from Africa to Europe.

Let us therefore look at some figures for North America up to December 1986 (Table 2.1). By the end of December 1986 there were over 28,000 cases of AIDS in the United States, more than half of whom were dead; one of the important points to make about AIDS is that at any one time about 50–55 per cent of those who have been diagnosed in any population will be dead.

Table 2.2: AIDS, United Kingdom, December 1986

	Total (Females in parenthesis)		Deaths
Homosexual/bisexual	538		244
Haemophiliac	25		19
Intravenous drug abuser	9	(2)	2
Homosexual/intravenous drug abuser	6		4
Blood recipient			
Abroad	6	(3)	5
UK	4	(1)	4
Heterosexual			
Abroad	14	(5)	9
UK	4	(3)	3
Child of positive mother	3	(2)	2
Other	1	(1)	1
Totals	610	(17)	293

The disease in North America is still principally one of men, although infected women are now beginning to appear. In this connection, particular attention should be paid to drug addicts. Drug addiction is commonly linked to prostitution, and is often financed by prostitution, which means that this is one of the important ways in which the virus may spread from the drug addict population into the non-addict groups.

Heterosexual transmission is also now occurring in North America outside the drug addiction group. But homosexual and bisexual men are still the groups most likely to contract the disease.

Figures for the United Kingdom up to December 1986 show 610 cases, of which 293 are dead (Table 2.2). In January 1987 there was a sudden increase — the figure rose sharply — and by the end of January it was almost 700. Very few females in this country appear to be infected, but drug abusers are a special risk and again homosexual and bisexual males are at the top of the list.

One of the tragic groups, of course, are the haemophiliacs, who became infected with this virus through no activity on their part. In the West Midlands area of the UK there are 260 HIV-positive patients and of these 141 are haemophiliacs.

As regards immunology, we refer to the virus as the antigen,

Table 2.3: HIV antibody-positive, December 1984/December 1986, England, Wales and Northern Ireland

	Male	Female	Total
Homosexual/bisexual	1964	—	1964
Haemophiliac/blood disorder	927	3	930
Intravenous drug abuser	148	69	217
Homosexual/intravenous drug abuser	14	—	14
Blood recipient	17	9	26
Heterosexual	10	38	48
Child of positive mother	5	4	9
Uncertain/unknown	635	34	669
Totals	3720	157	3877

and to the response of the immune system to the virus — i.e. the protein produced in response to the virus — as the antibody. Seroconversion is the appearance of the antibody in the blood, and for HIV disease this usually occurs about four to six weeks after infection, although it can take as long as three months (and occasionally even longer).

If we now consider HIV antibody-positive individuals reported between December 1984 (when testing started) and December 1986, in England, Wales and Northern Ireland, we find that almost 4,000 people are known to have been infected (Table 2.3). It has been suggested that this figure could be multiplied by 10, i.e. 4,000 known, but possibly a total pool of 40,000 infected, but such an estimate is, of course, pure conjecture.

Again it can be seen that the patterns of infection are fairly similar to those of AIDS itself. But one can see here the numbers of infected intravenous drug users rising. AIDS is still mainly a disease of the homosexual and the haemophiliac, but infected drug addicts are now unfortunately beginning to become more common. In Scotland, and especially in Edinburgh and Dundee, the problem with the drug addict is a particularly serious one.

On the subject of screening of blood donors, the figures show that among the first 2½ million donations tested there were very few positives (1 per 50,000 tested), and that those who were positive were nearly all men in high-risk groups and nearly all homosexual men. Sir Donald Acheson, Chief Medical Officer at the Department of Health and Social Security, has stated that the

16

Table 2.4: Acquired immune deficiency syndrome

---

1   A disease that is indicative of cellular immunodeficiency, e.g.
    Kaposi's sarcoma in a patient under the age of 60 or opportunistic
    infection.

2   No known cause of cellular immunodeficiency.

---

chances of catching AIDS from blood transfusions is probably about one in a million.

AIDS is often discussed without being defined, and it is worthwhile therefore setting out this brief definition of the disease (Table 2.4).

It should be noted that it is a cellular immune deficiency disease associated with two things, either opportunistic infections or the skin tumour, Kaposi's sarcoma.

The AIDS virus attacks certain targets in the body (Figure 2.1) and Table 2.5 lists the results of the cells being infected. In consequence the body's immune system may begin to wane — this being demonstrated first by an inability to cope with minor infections, then with serious infections, the development of the skin tumour and finally the invasion of the brain cells producing neurological or psychiatric illness or both.

One of the particularly worrying aspects of brain disease is that neurological and psychiatric illness can present in patients who have not yet developed AIDS. In other words their immune system is apparently still healthy, they have neither Kaposi's sarcoma nor infections, but brain disease presents *de novo*, antedating the immune deficiency. Although uncommon it has already occurred.

Figure 2.1: Areas of the body attacked by AIDS virus

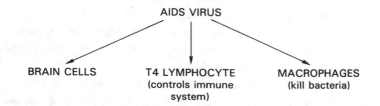

```
                        AIDS VIRUS



      BRAIN CELLS      T4 LYMPHOCYTE        MACROPHAGES
                       (controls immune     (kill bacteria)
                           system)
```

17

Table 2.5: HIV infection

Waning immune system
Minor infections
Serious infections
Skin tumour
(Kaposi's sarcoma)
Invasion of brain cells
Neurological illness
Psychiatric illness

What happens when a person is infected with the virus? What is the outcome? Initially there was conjecture as to whether the body might be able to eradicate the virus, but as Dr Weber has already pointed out, this is unlikely.

Follow-up of the disease is of only a five-year duration, and after five years it appeared that about one-third of those infected with AIDS would have the disease, one-third would have AIDS-related disorders (i.e. symptoms but not serious illness) some of whom will eventually go on to develop AIDS, and that one-third will remain healthy.

But these figures now appear to be changing. The Germans suggest that probably 50 per cent rather than 33 per cent of those affected will have AIDS after five years, and there are pessimists who propose that in possibly ten years' time the proportion may rise to 100 per cent — but that of course is speculation.

It does seem, however, that any group of HIV-infected individuals is, in a sense, like an iceberg, with those known to have AIDS being only the tip of it.

Turning now briefly to some of the symptoms and some of the clinical features of this disease: they vary from non-specific symptoms, such as weight loss, diarrhoea, or enlargement of the lymph glands, to much more serious conditions with opportunistic infections causing pneumonia or dementia.

The classical serious presentations of AIDS are: Kaposi's sarcoma or pneumonia caused by *Pneumocystis carinii*, the organism mentioned by Dr Weber.

With regard to the nervous system Dr Weber has mentioned the invasion of the CNS by this virus, and as a result of this invasion it seems likely that almost any neurological or psychiatric illness recognised to date may manifest as a symptom of HIV infection; some are listed here:

acute encephalopathy
chronic encephalopathy
acute meningitis
transverse myelitis
peripheral neuropathy
acute psychosis
chronic psychosis

Other neurological manifestations of AIDS include opportunistic infections such as toxoplasmosis and cryptococcosis, and cerebral lymphomas.

What is very fascinating is that certain of the opportunist organisms that cause serious infection in patients with AIDS, originate in animals. This is interesting because of course it is likely that the virus itself was a primate virus — a monkey virus — but how it escaped from monkey into man we do not know. But *Toxoplasma gondii*, the organism that causes brain disease in AIDS sufferers, is very common in domestic cats: another organism that creates a serious infection in AIDS patients is *Cryptosporidium*, which produces severe intractable and untreatable diarrhoea; it probably also originates in animals.

HOW IS AIDS TRANSMITTED

The virus is known to be present in the following fluids:

blood
seminal fluid
vaginal secretions
saliva
tears
breast milk

Possible salivary spread is one of the aspects of AIDS that creates a great deal of discussion, particularly in the press and on television.

There is no evidence, however, that saliva transmits the infection. Indeed, in patients who are infected by this virus there are antibodies to it in saliva, and I would suggest therefore that saliva is not a way in which this particular virus can be transmitted.

The ways in which it is transmitted are, of course, well known — sexually, by means of blood or blood products, and from mother to child — both the unborn child and possibly also the neonate. A child can be infected not only *in utero* but also during delivery, and possibly also from breast milk after the birth.

As to safety in the context of the Health Service and related staff, the fears are great.

As far as I know this statement published in the *British Medical Journal* of 15 March 1986 remains true today (27 February 1987):

'No health care worker has contracted AIDS from a patient.'

However there have been four episodes of seroconversion to HIV following deep needle-stick injury. By this I mean someone, a member of hospital staff, usually a nurse, has taken a needle out of an AIDS patient dripping with blood, tried to resheath it, missed the sheath and driven it into his or her hand. In effect, by so doing the person has given himself or herself a mini-transfusion of blood contaminated with the AIDS virus.

That is the bad news, but the good news is (and I only select one example) that very many health care staff, both in this country and in the United States, have been contaminated with blood from AIDS patients on their skin, or on mucous membranes and have not been infected. A study taken from the *Annals of Internal Medicine* (*104*, 644; 1986) shows that 150 health care workers who had looked after 238 patients, and who had had skin or mucous membrane contamination (the mucous membrane usually being the eyes) with infected blood, had no seroconversion.

Another reassuring report *New England Journal of Medicine*, 6 February 1986) is a household study of 101 non-sexual contacts of 39 AIDS patients in the United States. No seroconversion resulted, apart from the child born of an infected woman drug addict.

The same study lists some of the things these people shared with the AIDS patients within the home. It is not a highly infectious disease.

Another study (*Lancet*, 13 September 1986), of special interest to those who work in psychiatric hospitals where hepatitis B infection is prevalent, was undertaken in France, in a school where haemophiliac children were taught along with non-haemophiliacs. Half of the haemophiliacs were positive for HIV but none of the non-haemophiliacs. All of the haemophiliacs were positive for the hepatitis B virus and four of the non-haemophiliacs had contracted it. It would seem, therefore, that hepatitis B is more infectious than HIV, although the situation may be affected by the fact that the amount of hepatitis B virus in the blood of carriers is much greater than the amount of HIV. For practical purposes, therefore, when someone is known to be HIV-positive in hospital or in a clinic, similar precautions are taken to those that have been developed over the years for patients who are positive for hepatitis B.

The virus is not particularly hardy outside the body. It is destroyed by heat, $-65°F$; by a number of disinfectants; including hypochlorite, which is of course domestic bleach. It does not appear to survive very long once it has left the human body.

WHAT ABOUT CURES AND VACCINES?

Dr Weber has painted a gloomy picture. There are no cures, there are no vaccines. There are drugs available that will suppress the virus and the best known is a Burroughs Wellcome agent, AZT, now known as Zovidarine or Retrovir. AZT will suppress the virus in the human body and will pass the blood–brain barrier into the brain. It has side-effects associated with its use, and maybe as many as 40 per cent of patients who get it feel unwell while they are receiving it; and when the drug is stopped the virus comes back. It is not a cure; it is a suppressive agent.

Nevertheless, clinical trials with this drug are starting shortly in this country, and other drugs are in the pipeline. None of them, however, as far as I know, offer a cure.

21

Table 2.6: AIDS — new patients — United Kingdom

Actual		Predicted	
1979	2	1986	620
1980	0	1987	1440
1981	5	1988	3350
1982	19	1989	7750
1983	52	1990	18,030
1984	111		
1985	155		

It has been suggested that while the use of a viral suppressant agent may make the patient feel a bit better, and live longer, it may also actually increase the incidence of neuropsychiatric disease. In other words, one controls the virus in the periphery of the body but it goes on multiplying in the brain.

WHAT ABOUT A VACCINE?

This virus, as has been indicated elsewhere, is very complex, and the hopes for vaccines are still not particularly high, although there are some chinks of light in the darkness. For example, workers in Glasgow have developed a vaccine against the cat leukaemia virus which is also a retrovirus, and there is hope that further work may build on this achievement.

It must be borne in mind, however, that even if a vaccine became available next week it would have no use at all in the management of those already infected. It would only be of value to prevent infection in the future.

So what about the future? In the United States this prediction has been made: by 1991 a total of 145,000 AIDS patients (these are not HIV-positive, these are AIDS patients). It has been estimated, incidentally, that in New York City there are 200,000 drug addicts, 100,000 of them currently infected with the virus.

And what about this country? The figures in Table 2.6 were produced towards the end of 1986: actual cases being shown on the left, predicted cases on the right. The prediction was 620 for 1986, and it was very close to the actual figure, which was 610. Mathematical models predict for 1990 over 18,000 cases —

Figure 2.2: The AIDS iceberg (from *Nature*, 6 November 1986)

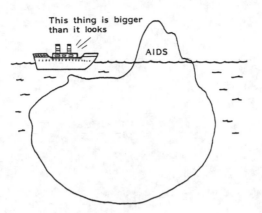

again of AIDS — and not of HIV infection — for this country, unless a cure is found, or the risk groups — and that of course means all of us — modify our sexual behaviour.

This final illustration (Figure 2.2) is taken from *Nature*, and it illustrates very clearly that the patients suffering from AIDS — approximately 700 in this country — are but the tip of the iceberg. Below the surface there are many, many others who are infected and will eventually go on to develop the disease.

3

Psychiatric Sequelae of HIV

James W. Dilley

As the Director of the AIDS Health Project at the University of California, San Francisco (UCSF), a mental health promotion and AIDS risk reduction programme of the San Francisco Department of Public Health and the Department of Psychiatry, UCSF, I have had considerable experience with the variety of problems that can be seen by the practising psychiatrist.

Let me begin by clarifying that I am using the title 'Psychiatric Sequelae of the Human Immunodeficiency Virus' to refer not only to those syndromes which can be directly attributed to HIV infection itself, but also to those disorders in personal functioning that are more indirectly related to the threat of infection with this virus. I want to begin with some general remarks about the role of psychiatry and mental health professionals in the AIDS epidemic, and then move on to discuss functional disorders in those at risk. I will conclude my remarks with a discussion of the neuropsychiatric complications seen in those with HIV infection.

During the first few years of this decade, AIDS has emerged as a growing public health menace around the world. With this realisation has come not only the awareness that a deadly, previously unknown and untreatable disease has thrust itself abruptly on the public consciousness, but also that the sense of security from disease, and the faith in modern medical science to protect us from it, have been eroded.

We have been forced to watch as young, vibrant, and

previously healthy members of society are suddenly and inexplicably being brought down. Archetypal images of sweeping pestilence and fear of death, have consequently emerged in the public awareness. These images in the Western world have usually been associated with far-away, exotic places that we watched safely, at a distance, as footage on the evening news.

With AIDS, however, we have suddenly been faced with the realisation that these far-away exotic places are not so far away and not so exotic. The deserts of Ethiopia have been replaced with the Victorian row houses of San Francisco, the bustling streets of Manhattan, and the capitals of Europe.

The world now watches as the numbers of diagnosed cases and the numbers of dead and dying steadily increase. Magical thinking occurs on a grand scheme as millions of people turn a deaf ear towards the educational messages that have begun to come forth.

And why shouldn't they? Which of us is not prone to rationalising unpleasantness? Bad things happen to others — not to ourselves. Which of us does not occasionally feel the regressive tug of dependent fantasies, wherein we don't have to accept responsibility for taking care of ourselves, but can instead leave it to someone — the doctor — or something — science and technology — to take care of everything for us.

Sexually transmitted diseases in the 1980s have either been seen as chronic and irritating, like herpes, or as something to be momentarily embarrassed about, treated and forgotten. AIDS has changed all of that.

The spectre of AIDS then, raises a number of issues that are at once both very old and very new to the mental health practitioner. For example, the issues of death and dying have, of course, always been with us. The need to face the fact that large numbers of young people in their prime are dying from a communicable disease which we are unable to treat, is new. Issues of sexuality have always been with us but the need to address these issues publicly and in explicit terms is unprecedented.

These are the kinds of issues that mental health professionals have experience in confronting. Helping others to adjust to trouble in their lives, to cope with loss and to adapt to the need to make changes in the way an individual's life is led are not new challenges to mental health professionals. AIDS has brought these issues to the fore for millions around the world. The mental health practitioner, bringing his or her experience in dealing with these kinds of issues, can be helpful in the struggle against this disease.

Furthermore, because AIDS is primarily transmitted by specific high-risk sexual activities, and by the sharing of infected needles, AIDS is a disease of *behaviour*. As such, it falls squarely within the purview of psychiatry. Because AIDS, at present, is largely a disease of socially disenfranchised groups and because issues of stigma and prejudice compound the emotional distress of patients facing a life-threatening illness, the mental health professional has an obligation to intervene.

Finally, because AIDS is first and foremost a medical illness with complex brain–behaviour relationships, psychiatrists, who are physicians as well as specialists in the behavioural sciences, bring special knowledge, skills and talents to the treatment of people with the disease.

AIDS-RELATED PSYCHIATRIC DISORDERS

Let me now turn to a discussion of the continuum of AIDS-related psychiatric disorders. Figure 3.1 summarises the range of disorders that can be seen in the group of patients most concerned about this disease.

The spectrum of AIDS-related psychiatric disorders covers the range of anxiety and depressive disorders. To these should be added panic disorder and hypochondriasis or somatisation disorder. These latter conditions are generally seen in conjunction with significant anxiety or depression but are classified as distinct disorders. The point should be made here that, for people with AIDS-related conditions, these kinds of problems are even more in evidence than among people with AIDS.

Two prospective longitudinal studies, one in New York and one in San Francisco, are studying the psychosocial aspects of AIDS. Both have shown that people with AIDS-related conditions

27

Figure 3.1: The continuum of AIDS-related psychiatric problems. Problems manifesting themselves primarily in anxiety symptoms are shown above, while those predominantly affective are shown below the arrow

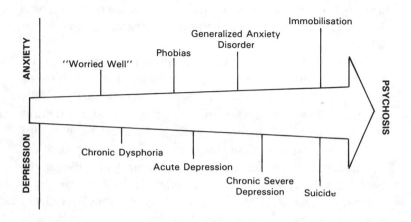

(ARC) report higher levels of distress than patients diagnosed with AIDS. The most common explanation for this finding is that 'life in the Grey Zone', i.e. not knowing what is happening to one's health and constantly living with the spectre of developing AIDS, is more unsettling than actually knowing that one has the full-blown disease.

Other important factors are that these patients are sometimes not granted the same legitimate sick role by their social support system as people with AIDS, and, in the US, they may be ineligible for social programmes whose services they need because they do not have a diagnosis that is always recognised as serious.

Patients with hypochondriasis or somatisation disorder are often homosexual or bisexual men who believe themselves to be infected with the virus. These men are hypervigilant, chronically distressed and constantly surveying their bodies for signs or symptoms of what they believe is the inevitability of an AIDS diagnosis.

For those patients who present with high levels of anxiety and distress, but who have little objective reason for their concern— for example, a homosexual man with one unsafe sexual encounter who obsesses continually and is unable to be reassured, or the heterosexual married man who paid for sex at a brothel and now is beset by worries that he is infected — a recommendation in favour of antibody testing may be useful.

The many issues raised by antibody testing are complex and beyond the scope of this chapter. However, in the instance of the cases just described, testing may be therapeutic as long as the testing experience occurs within the context of an ongoing psychotherapeutic relationship. This ensures that the results can then be discussed and understood in relation to the larger issues in the patients' life. Little formal evaluation of these patients can be found in literature at present, but clinical reports confirm that these 'AIDS anxiety syndrome' patients are growing in number.

It should also be appreciated, however, that the presenting complaints, which focus on the fear of AIDS, usually evolve over time and appear to be the consequence of displacement in which other characterological conflicts are displaced on to the fear of AIDS. Psychotherapy, sometimes in conjunction with appropriate anti-anxiety or anti-depressant medications, is indicated for these patients.

Finally, it should be stressed that the patient's symptoms will frequently persist despite the assurance of a negative test. The images of becoming sick with AIDS often persist and serve a self-flagellating, or self-defeating function related to underlying personality issues. Nevertheless, mutual knowledge of a negative test helps to anchor both the therapist and the patient in the security that the fears and the distress experienced, while certainly real, are appropriately in the realm of psychological concerns.

ADAPTATION FOR THE 'WORRIED WELL'

The 'worried well' is a term that has come to be applicable to nearly every informed sexually active person. Originally used to refer to homosexual and bisexual men who were physically healthy but worried about their possibility of becoming infected, the term has taken a larger meaning as greater numbers of people outside the primary risk groups become ill.

29

The facts of the situation are such that for sexually active homosexual or bisexual men or intravenous drug users, a certain level of fear is to be expected and acknowledged. In San Francisco, for example, where solid epidemiological estimates of the seroprevalence of HIV infection among homosexual men approached 60 per cent, a healthy fear is adaptive and may lead to a positive change in high-risk behaviour. The issue of making and maintaining a positive adaptation is one in which psychiatry can and should be helpful.

A model for this adaptation is seen in Figure 3.2. This illustration serves well as a visual representation of the kinds of strategies employed at the AIDS Health Project, University of California, San Francisco. Collaboratively designed by a group of mental health practitioners who were faced daily by the concerns of scores of patients struggling to cope with the demands for behaviour change placed on them by the AIDS epidemic, the Project employs a psychologically sophisticated approach to the complexities of establishing and maintaining major behavioural changes. Any change programme is facilitated by peer support and social connectedness, sense of mastery, and education.

In considering these issues further, it is worth noting a study undertaken in San Francisco early in 1985 by Coates and others. The study documented sexual behaviour changes among homosexual men, and also asked those who had not made changes consistent with the guidelines for low-risk behaviour, why they had not done so. Their results highlighted three beliefs among the men who had not made changes.

First, the men who continued to engage in high-risk behaviour stated that they simply didn't believe in AIDS or that it could actually be spread sexually. Homosexual men have long been accustomed to authorities of various kinds telling them not to have sex.

Second, those who had made no changes felt that there was no support in the homosexual community for making these kinds of changes. Thus, to do so would mean that they would be ostracised and alienated from their community. Or, stated another way, high-risk sexual behaviour was felt to be an expected and necessary activity if one were to be accepted by one's peers.

Figure 3.2: An integrated model for psychiatry's positive potential roles in meeting the mental health challenges of AIDS

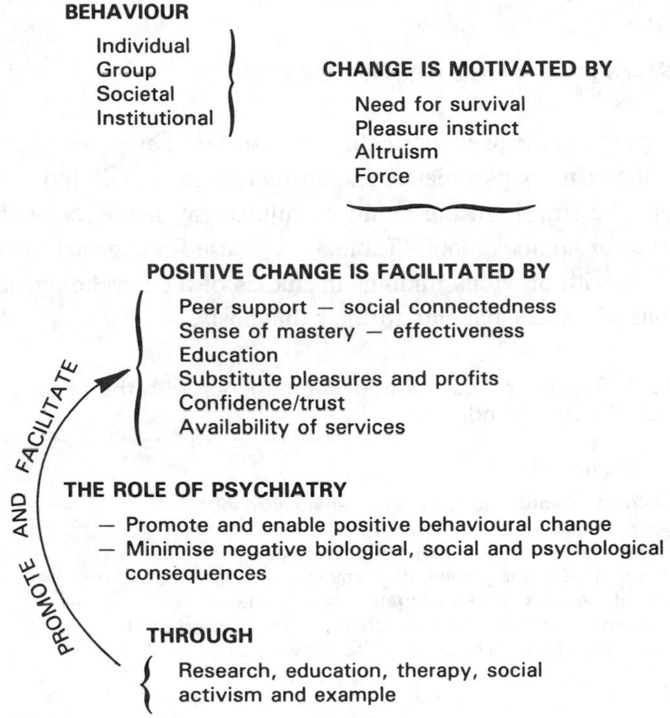

BEHAVIOUR

Individual
Group
Societal
Institutional

CHANGE IS MOTIVATED BY

Need for survival
Pleasure instinct
Altruism
Force

POSITIVE CHANGE IS FACILITATED BY

Peer support — social connectedness
Sense of mastery — effectiveness
Education
Substitute pleasures and profits
Confidence/trust
Availability of services

THE ROLE OF PSYCHIATRY

— Promote and enable positive behavioural change
— Minimise negative biological, social and psychological consequences

PROMOTE AND FACILITATE

THROUGH

Research, education, therapy, social activism and example

The third and last belief that differentiated the men who had not made sexual behaviour changes was that they reported a lower social skill level than those men who had successfully made changes. These men felt they simply 'couldn't do it'; they felt they didn't have the skill or capacity to discuss a potential sexual encounter and place limits on the kinds of activities to be engaged in before the encounter took place. Thus, these men felt helpless and largely at the mercy of their partner and their own impulses.

These are the kind of issues, then, which can be problematic for homosexual men who are contemplating the need to make changes in behaviour. Mental health practitioners can be a great help both in understanding the complexities of behavioural change and in working for programmes that will support and train individuals in making lifestyle changes. The AIDS Health Project is concerned with both these issues.

NEUROPSYCHIATRIC DISORDERS

Turning now to the psychiatric disorders suffered by people with AIDS, the primary psychiatric diagnostic categories fall into two groups. The first is in the realm of adjustment disorders, with depressed or anxious mood (Table 3.1). These findings are very consistent with previous findings in studies of the psychological reactions of cancer patients to their diagnosis.

Table 3.1: Psychiatric consultations in patients with the acquired immunodeficiency syndrome (AIDS)

Frequent diagnoses
- Adjustment disorder (depressed or anxious mood)
- Major depression
- Delirium (narcotics, steroids, fever, hypoxia)
- Dementia (AIDS encephalopathy, toxoplasmosis, progressive multifocal leukoencephalopathy, lymphoma)
- Treatment-related side-effects (chemotherapy, interferon)
- Previous psychiatric illness or personality disorder

In addition to having to come to terms with the usual existential searching that accompanies the diagnosis of a life-threatening illness and the potential for stigmatisation that is so common with this disease, the person with AIDS must also cope with the anticipatory grieving that comes with facing a limited life expectancy. The expected multiple losses are constant psychic companions and can result in waves of emotion as the individual learns to live with the reality of the diagnosis.

As our understanding of AIDS has progressed, however, a new psychosocial stressor has emerged to confront the person with AIDS. This new stressor is being promulgated in part by the media, as vividly demonstrated by this headline from the *San Francisco Examiner*, 'The AIDS That Kills the Mind: Terrifying Symptoms of Mental Deterioration'. Headlines of this sort are inflammatory and cause a good deal of anxiety among people with AIDS.

Let me now turn to a brief review of what is known about the neuropsychiatric complications in AIDS.

Evolving research has shown that in addition to the opportunistic diseases that can strike the central nervous system of people with AIDS, there are also degenerative neuropathological changes that occur as a result of the virus itself. These pathological changes can occur in the brain and spinal cord, and may eventually result in changes in thinking, feeling and behaviour as the machinery of the brain begins to function in a less efficient manner. These changes are of particular importance to the mental health professional who may be the first person to notice or be notified of them.

It is also important to keep in mind that a person with AIDS, like any other medically ill population of patients, is prey to a variety of problems that can result in altered mental status. However, the most important causes of mental status change for the purposes of this chapter can be found summarised in Table 3.2.

This table summarises the neurological complications of the first 352 patients with AIDS treated at the University of California, San Francisco. Of particular importance are the non-viral syndromes, particularly toxoplasmosis, a parasitic infection of the brain, and *Cryptococcus* a fungus that can also cause central nervous system dysfunction. These infections are particularly important for the mental health care professional because they are very treatable illnesses. Thus, those who work with patients in an outpatient setting in particular should be familiar with the common presenting complaints of patients with these disorders. These are summarised below:

Toxoplasmosis encephalitis
 Presentation:
  Confusion, lethargy 50 per cent
  Seizures 30 per cent
  Motor impairment 20 per cent

 Majority have fever, chills or anorexia
 Onset may be sudden or indolent

Table 3.2: Neurological complications in AIDS spectrum patients

CNS disease	Percentage	Known medical treatment
A. *Viral syndromes*		
Atypical aseptic meningitis	7	None
Herpes simplex encephalitis	3	Arachidonic acid or acyclovir
Progressive multifocal leukoencephalopathy	2	Possibly arachidonic acid
AIDS dementia	?	None
B. *Non-viral syndromes*		
Toxoplasma gondii	32	Pyrimethamine and sulphadiazine
Cryptococcus neoformans	13	Amphotericin B and 5-flurocytosine
Candida albicans	2	Amphotericin B and ? 5-flurocytosine
Atypical *Mycobacteria*	2	INH, ethambutol and rifampin
Other	2	
C. *Neoplasms*	10	
Primary CNS lymphoma	5	Radiation therapy
CNS and systemic lymphoma	4	Radiation therapy and chemotherapy
Kaposi's sarcoma	1	Radiation therapy and chemotherapy
D. *Cerebrovascular accidents*	3	Treat aetiology
Endocarditis		
Herpes zoster arteritis		
Idiopathic thrombocytopenia		
E. *Neuropathies, myopathy*	?	
Distal symmetrical neuropathy		Amitriptyline
Chronic inflammatory polyneuropathy		Consider plasmapheresis
Vacuolar myelopathy		
F. *Metabolic and systemic changes*	?	Treat aetiology
Hypoxia secondary to *Pneumocystis carinii* pneumonia		
Electrolyte imbalance		
Nutritional deficiencies		

Adapted from: Levy, Bredeson, and Rosenblum (1985). 'Neurological manifestations of AIDS', *Journal of Neurosurgery*, *62*, 475–495.

Cryptococcus meningitis

Presentation: fever, headaches, meningeal signs
Onset: usually sudden

Toxoplasmosis is treated successfully in more than 85 per cent of patients. Improvement usually occurs within one or two weeks with treatment continuing for life. Cognitive changes that may have been the result of the infection will sometimes show dramatic improvement with almost complete recovery to normal mentation. Treatment for *Cryptococcus* is not quite as good but improvement is to be expected.

How extensive is the problem of neuropsychiatric complications in AIDS? Most studies report that between 30 and 75 per cent of patients with AIDS develop neurological complications that include, though are certainly not limited to, the kinds of behavioural problems that will be discussed here. Also, as mentioned previously, a variety of autopsy reports on patients with AIDS have shown that as many as 90 per cent of brains at autopsy show pathological changes. Additionally, between 10 and 25 per cent of patients who develop AIDS can show neurological changes as their presenting problem.

Evidence for primary brain infection by human immunodeficiency virus (HIV)

While an increased incidence of encephalopathy had been noted among hospitalised patients with AIDS from very early in the epidemic, the understanding that this finding was due, in part, to primary infection by HIV did not occur until early to mid-1985.

The first significant report on this subject was in January of 1985 when Shaw reported isolating HIV from the brains of five patients at autopsy. In a companion article in the same issue of the journal *Science*, Gonda and colleagues discussed the genomic relationship between HIV and a well-known member of the lentivirus family, the Visna virus. This virus, one of the 'slow viruses' known to cause a degenerative neurological disease in sheep, was shown to be structurally very similar to HIV.

35

This indirect evidence further supported the hypothesis that the degree and frequency of neurological impairment in this group of patients was probably a consequence of HIV infection itself.

A few months later, at the First International Conference on AIDS in Atlanta, Georgia, Dr Gajdusek of the National Cancer Institute, a well-known researcher for his work on Jakob–Creutzfeldt disease, another slow viral disease, presented the first experimental evidence in chimpanzees that the virus introduced peripherally could later be found in the central nervous system.

In this study, Gajdusek and others took biopsy specimens from the brains of patients with AIDS who had encephalopathy prior to death. The biopsy material was then put into solution, placed into a syringe and injected into the peripheral veins of a group of chimpanzees. After several weeks, brain biopsies were performed on the chimps and HIV was isolated from the specimens. This was the first demonstration that the virus, though introduced into the body peripherally, could penetrate the blood–brain barrier and reside in the brain.

Since these experiments, a large literature now exists on various aspects of the neurological problems in AIDS including the clinical findings in children with this disease.

Clinical manifestations of nervous system involvement

Given the known affinity for nervous tissue of HIV, one would expect a degree of neurological impairment in children infected with the virus similar to that seen in adults. Though little has been published to date on this issue, Leon Epstein and his colleagues at the New Jersey Medical School recently published an important article on the neurological problems of children with AIDS. In this study, 38 children who had been infected with HIV for periods ranging from two months to four years were followed prospectively for an average of 19 months. Twenty of the 38 children were diagnosed with AIDS (Table 3.3).

Of the 38 children in the study, 28 developed some kind of progressive dementia or stable encephalopathy during the study

Table 3.3: Clinical staging of human immunodeficiency virus infection and neurological dysfunction*

Clinical stage	Progressive encepha-lopathy	Static encepha-lopathy	Normal
AIDS	16	4	0
AIDS-related complex	3	3	6
Asymptomatic†	1	0	2

* Results are expressed as numbers of children.
† Immunologically asymptomatic but seropositive for human immunodeficiency virus.

Table 3.4: Neurological findings of progressive encephalopathy

	No. of patients with finding	Total no. of patients
Loss of developmental milestones or subcortical dementia	19	20
Impaired brain growth	19	20
Secondary microcephaly	12	20
Cortical atrophy on CT scan*	14	16
Generalized weakness with pyramidal signs	19	20
Pseudobulbar palsy†	6	16
Ataxia‡	4	8
Seizures	5	20
Myoclonus	2	20
Extrapyramidal rigidity	3	20

* Computed tomographic (CT) scans obtained in 16 patients only.
† Not reliably evaluated in infants less than 12 months of age.
‡ Evaluated only in children who achieved independent ambulation.

period. Of particular note in this regard is the seropositive asymptomatic child. This child, though free of any overt physical symptoms of disease indicating a diagnosis of AIDS or AIDS-related complex (ARC), nevertheless displayed behavioural problems consistent with a diagnosis of progressive encephalopathy.

How then did these children look clinically and what kinds of problems did they display? As can be seen from Table 3.4, one of the most common findings in children with HIV infection is the loss of developmental milestones. In addition, 19 of the 20 children with AIDS showed evidence of impaired brain growth as measured by findings of cortical atrophy on computerised tomograms (CT scans), and/or secondary microcephaly. Generalised weakness, extrapyramidal signs and other indications of motor problems are also seen. This predilection for neuromuscular disorders is also consistent with clinical findings in adult patients with AIDS.

CLINICAL FINDINGS IN ADULT PATIENTS

In adult patients with AIDS, the extent of neuropathological changes seen at autopsy is widespread and consistent with the global cognitive changes seen during life. Thus, in a sample of 26 patients with subacute encephalitis whose brains were examined post-mortem by David Ho at the Massachusetts General Hospital in Boston, 20 of the 26 (77 per cent) had subacute encephalitis without superimposed lesions due to opportunistic infections and/or lymphoma. Lesions of subacute encephalitis were predominantly distributed in:

cerebral cortex	85 per cent
white matter	92 per cent
frontal lobes	56 per cent
temporal lobes	67 per cent
basal ganglia	76 per cent
amygdala	78 per cent
hippocampus	62 per cent

Thus, widespread areas of the brain can be affected by HIV.

In addition to a variety of areas in the brain that can be affected, a number of different cell types are also involved. Astrocytes, oligodendrocytes, macrophages and multinucleated giant cells have all been shown to be infected with the virus in these patients. This process is demonstrated in Figure 3.3, which shows an electron micrograph of HIV particles budding from the surface of a macrophage taken from the brain of a patient with AIDS (National Cancer Institute).

In addition, researchers at the University of California, San Diego, have also shown that endothelial cells of brain capillaries can be infected. These cells, of course, maintain the integrity of the capillary and their infection by the virus may play a role in the development of the dementing disorders seen in AIDS.

The pathological mechanism for the development of the brain disorders in AIDS is not yet fully understood. One theory is that because of the endothelial cell involvement and the local inflammatory processes that occur, the changes in brain function that result are due to these inflammatory processes that cause the endothelial cells of the capillaries to leak. This leakage results in the collection of oedema which compresses the brain tissue and causes dysfunction. Supporting this possibility is the cognitive deficits seen in patients who receive radiation therapy for brain tumours. In these patients, organic brain syndromes may occur strictly on the basis of cerebral oedema.

Other possible mechanisms for the underlying cause of the brain dysfunction seen in these patients are that the infected macrophages or the virus itself may secrete some toxic substance which is responsible for the destruction of brain tissue or, some other, as yet unidentified factor may be responsible.

The clinical findings in adult AIDS patients with neuropsychiatric complications fall into three general categories. These are cognitive, behavioural and motor problems and a further description of each can be seen summarised in Tables 3.5 and 3.6.

The earliest manifestations of the dementia seen in these patients are personality changes or memory loss, particularly delayed memory loss.

For example, in a group of 22 AIDS patients referred for psychiatric consultation at San Francisco General Hospital we studied the differences between short term memory impairment and delayed memory loss. We found that while only 23 per cent of our sample demonstrated short term memory loss, 68 per cent had delayed memory loss. Delayed memory is defined as 30 minutes or longer. These data strongly suggest that the standard bedside mental status examination is really insufficient to pick up this kind of early cognitive change in these patients.

Another issue that is particularly relevant to the practising mental health practitioner is that AIDS patients will frequently present in the early stages of HIV neuropsychological disorders

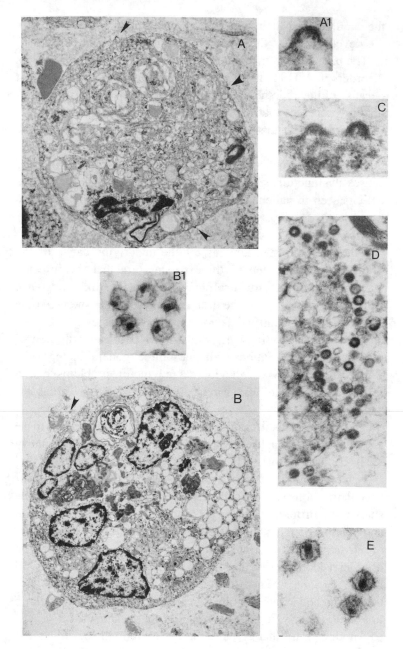

Figure 3.3: Transmission electron micrographs of tissue from a patient. Typical virus-producing (A) mononuclear cells (× 9300) and (B) multinucleated cells (× 5000) rich in lipids, myelin fibres, and viral particles in varying stages of maturation, are shown. Three particles are budding from the surface of the mononuclear cell (A, arrows); the upper one is enlarged (A1). Two are budding from another cell (C). Late budding and free immature particles with ring-shaped nucleoids are abundant (D). The nucleoids in most mature virions are tangentially or perpendicularly sectioned (B and B1) and only occasional longitudinally sectioned particles showing the conical core shell are seen (E). The outer membrane of the mature virions is usually deformed (B1 and E). (A1, B1, C, and E × 100,000; D × 50,000). At autopsy, fresh tissue samples were fixed in 2.5 per cent glutaraldehyde in phosphate-buffered saline. They were postfixed in 1 per cent OsO_4 dehydrated through graded ethanol, cleared in propylene oxide, and embedded in plastic. Thin sections were stained with uranyl acetate and lead citrate and examined on a Zeiss EM 10H.

Source: "Detection of AIDS virus in Macrophages in Brain from AIDS Patients with Encephalopathy", Koenig, S., *et al.*, *Science*, Vol. 233, pp. 1089–93, 5 September 1986. Reproduced with permission.

Table 3.5: The early manifestations of AIDS dementia

Symptoms
Cognitive
    Memory loss (names, historical details, appointments)
    Impaired concentration (lose track of conversation or reading)
    Mental slowing ('not as quick', less verbal, loss of spontaneity)
    Confusion (time or person)
Behavioural
    Apathy, withdrawal, 'depression'
    Agitation, confusion, hallucinations
Motor
    Unsteady gait
    Bilateral leg weakness
    Loss of co-ordination, impaired handwriting
    Tremor

Signs
Mental status examination
    Psychomotor slowing
    Impaired serial 7s or recent memory tasks
    'Normal' bedside examination
    Organic psychosis
Neurological examination
    Impaired rapid movements
    Gait ataxia (impaired tandem gait, rapid turns)
    Leg weakness
    Hyperreflexia
    Tremor
    Dysarthria
    Impaired smooth pursuit eye movements
Laboratory findings
    CSF: May show increase in protein and lymphocytes; normal or low glucose
    CT, MRI: May show cortical atrophy and ventricular enlargement

Adapted from: Navia and Price (1986) *Psychiatric Annals, 16*, 158–66 (March)

Table 3.6: The late manifestations of AIDS dementia

Symptoms
Cognitive
    Global dementia, confusion, distractibility, delayed verbal responses

Behavioural
    Vacant stare, restlessness, disinhibition, organic psychosis

Motor
    Slowing, truncal ataxia
    Weakness: legs > arms
    Pyramidal track signs: spasticity, hyperreflexia, tremor

Additional neurosigns
    Myoclonus
    Seizures
    Incontinence

Laboratory findings
    CT, MRI: showing cortical atrophy and white matter changes

---

Adapted from: Navia and Price (1986) *Psychiatric Annals, 16,* 158–66 (March)

with psychomotor retardation. This general slowing can very easily be confused with and misinterpreted as, a psychological response to the illness. In addition, impaired concentration, apathy, withdrawal, lassitude and fatigue can all be easily interpreted as psychological depression. When patients are agitated, confused or hallucinating, on the other hand, the diagnosis is more clear.

Finally, the use of laboratory tests is important though not always helpful. When tests are positive, such as the demonstration of a toxoplasmosis lesion on CT scan, they can be extremely important and allow for the institution of definitive treatment. However, if the CT scan is negative, it is less helpful because 25 per cent of patients with the infection can show a normal scan.

Another finding that is helpful and fairly common among these patients is cortical atrophy. However, the degree of atrophy may not be significant and may then be difficult to differentiate from that percentage of the normal population who show cortical atrophy.

Thus, the changes that can occur in the AIDS or HIV dementia complex are non-specific. Formal cognitive testing may be the best early indicator that something is wrong. In later stages of the illness the dementia complex may progress, resulting in a global dementia that affects all spheres. Patients can become mute and staring, and demonstrate a marked indifference to their surroundings and circumstances. Eventually coma and death may develop as the dementia progresses.

It should also be noted that while these kinds of problems are much more common among people with AIDS, they can also be seen in those with AIDS-related complex. Because of this development, the Centres for Disease Control have added this situation to the list of AIDS diagnoses.

Differentiating neuropsychiatric disorders from functional disorders

Given that many of the symptoms of neuropsychiatric dysfunction in AIDS can mimic the kinds of symptoms seen in functional disorders, the clinician must try to distinguish between them. The differential diagnosis for a patient presenting with a depressed mood must include organic affective disorder, in which the affective disturbance is thought to be a direct pathophysiological consequence of an identifiable cause (for example, HIV infection), and affective disorders in which the depressed mood is thought to be in reaction to the illness.

One important consideration in this regard is the natural history of the illness. For example, an affective disturbance in a newly diagnosed patient with Kaposi's sarcoma is more likely to be functional rather than as a consequence of primary brain infection by HIV. This patient's immune system is still relatively unimpaired. Thus, the clinician's index of suspicion is weighted toward interpreting the affective disorder as more likely due to a functional disorder, most commonly an adjustment disorder with depressed mood. As the patient moves along the trajectory of illness, however, and has had two or three bouts of pneumocystis, the likelihood that his presenting symptoms are explained at least in part by HIV infection is increased.

A second important consideration is the psychiatric history of the patient. For those with a history of major depression, or those with a family history of affective illness, the chances of these problems recurring are high, especially in the light of the stresses of coping with this disease.

As significant depression can occur with or without other cognitive signs, anti-depressant medication can be a useful adjunct in treatment. Focusing on the cognitive and affective aspects of depression can be helpful in determining the degree of depression present. Items such as low self-esteem, crying spells, ruminative suicidal thinking and social withdrawal are more important than the usual vegetative signs of depression which are likely to be related to the patients' underlying medical problems.

If the decision is made to treat the depression with anti-depressant medication, I recommend using drugs with low anti-cholinergic side-effects. Desipramine, imipramine and most recently, alprazolam have been used with fair success in these patients. The choice of low-anticholinergic medications is based on the assumption that the drying of mucous membranes common in medications with high-anticholinergic activity may foster the growth of candidiasis in the oropharynx. Additionally, it is well known that patients with pre-existing organic brain disorders are sensitive to the central effects of anticholinergic medications and may become increasingly confused and disoriented when placed on these drugs.

A similar comment should be made about the treatment of organic psychoses in patients with AIDS and the use of low anti-cholinergic psychotropic medications such as Haldol or Navane should be the drugs of choice.

Finally, it should be noted that these patients tend to be much more sensitive to medication effects in general, and should be monitored carefully. Severe extrapyramidal reactions have been noted and these patients should be treated with the lowest dose possible.

4

Medical and Psychiatric Nursing Care in the Department of Sexually Transmitted Diseases

Ben Thomas

This chapter is based on a discussion which took place between the members of a working group that looked specifically at the services for patients suffering with acquired immune deficiency syndrome/HIV and related conditions, attending the Department of Sexually Transmitted Diseases (STD Clinic) and associated inpatient units.

In the description an attempt is made to focus the broad-ranging content of the discussion on the service aspects, policies and procedures associated with AIDS/HIV and related conditions. The chapter follows subheadings which had previously been devised to concentrate on the psychosocial implications of AIDS/HIV and related conditions as they affect various components of the health and social services. Despite the differing aspects of the services required by these patients there are a number of recurring issues.

The working group included practitioners from various sections of the health and social services in the United Kingdom, was chaired by Mr John Tait, Principal Nursing Officer, DHSS, and the opening discussant was Dr Tom McManus, Consultant in Genito-Urinary Medicine, Camberwell Health Authority, King's College Hospital, London.

Although the majority of AIDS cases in the Camberwell Health Authority areas have presented initially to STD clinics, latterly an increasing number of patients with AIDS are presenting to their general practitioners, accident and emergency units, outpatient departments, and to medical and surgical wards in district general hospitals.

While this disease has previously been of specialist interest, it has now become the concern of general practitioners and all hospital and community workers. There is a need for good liaison and communication between these departments, and for all those concerned with the management of AIDS to have an adequate knowledge of the disease.

Since many of the signs and symptoms of AIDS are common to other diagnoses, and patients suffering with HIV may develop a wide spectrum of other diseases, it is particularly important for AIDS to be borne in mind by all disciplines who play a part in patient management.

This requires a sound knowledge of the possible range of the syndrome, and a knowledge of the most common presentations. Such information should prevent a diagnosis being missed.

It is important that these patients be well received in the initial stages of contact with the health and social services — i.e. be accepted in a sensitive and non-judgemental manner. Patients who receive counselling in preparation for HIV antibody testing seem better able to accept the result than those who do not receive such counselling.

However, it is clear that patients suffering with AIDS and related conditions have very special needs, since the diagnosis has far-reaching effects into all aspects of the patients' lives. Some patients may need psychiatric assessment: anxiety, depression and high suicidal risk being among the problems so far encountered.

The profound implications for the patients diagnosed as having AIDS mean that there is need for encouragement and support from a wide variety of disciplines within the health care structure. At the moment, however, there are serious deficiencies in the provision made to meet the psychological needs of these patients because of lack of resources and the prevailing negative attitudes of many health-care workers.

A newly diagnosed AIDS patient may receive an initial period of hospitalisation in order to complete diagnostic tests (e.g. admission to a surgical ward for lymph node biopsy), and/or to provide treatment for presenting infections. This period may vary, according to the severity of the symptoms. Ideally where possible, patients who have AIDS or HIV-related illnesses should be cared for at home, but the hospital needs to provide open access for any sudden deterioration in the clinical conditions.

A good inpatient service is required which should act as a 'safety-net'. The number and allocation of hospital beds devoted to AIDS-related disease is a matter of health district policy. The location of the beds is a matter for discussion.

Policies and procedures for medical nursing, psychiatric aspects of nursing, the clinical psychologist's work, and the role of the social services and voluntary agencies:
A number of specialist units are now in existence throughout the country. The units range from specialist wards in general hospitals to voluntarily run hospices. Different units each have a contribution to make, and the needs of the AIDS sufferer should ultimately dictate the most appropriate place in which care should be provided.

The situation which presently exists, whereby AIDS patients are nursed in random side-rooms throughout general hospitals, is unsatisfactory. It is appreciated that the principles of source isolation and protective isolation have to be applied when appropriate, but patients who are not at risk themselves, or at risk to other patients, need not be nursed separately, and the risks of depression, withdrawal and exclusion need continually to be emphasised.

Where patients are nursed in isolation, nurses should be allowed to spend as much time with them as possible, if required by the patient; and visitors should be encouraged to give emotional support and voluntary services, e.g. the Terrence Higgins Trust 'Buddy Volunteer Service', should be made welcome.

No structured approach to the care of AIDS patients at home exists in this country at present. Many AIDS sufferers who return home after discharge from hospital have to depend on relatives and friends to provide them with the care that they may require.

It is suggested that there is a need for a hospital-based ward or hospice nursing service, which would allow nurses to visit the patients at home when necessary. The system envisaged would be similar to the Macmillan nurses who have established this way of working with terminal cancer patients.

Wherever patients with AIDS/HIV infection are cared for, the health-care workers concerned should provide a service of maximum efficiency, linking inpatient and outpatient facilities. Close co-ordination is needed between medical staff and nursing and ancillary staff. Where possible continuity of care should be carried out, which may involve nurses moving from the ward to the outpatients department, and to the patient's home. This requires that hospital policies regarding admission and follow-up are clearly defined in advance. Such arrangements place a tremendous burden on these health-care workers, and their own need for support in meeting these responsibilities is considerable.

The innumerable challenges with which AIDS patients present nurses is also a major topic of debate. The skills demanded of the nurse caring for the AIDS patient are many and varied, and may include experience in high-dependency nursing, psychiatric nursing, care of the dying, prevention of cross-infection and experience with STD patients.

There is a general view that the nursing of AIDS patients is mainly the concern of general nurses, since AIDS patients may be suffering from a variety of symptoms requiring physical nursing care. However, it is recognised that a deficiency in the education of general nurses exists, in the areas of the interpersonal and counselling skills which this particular group of patients requires.

On the other hand, while it is unlikely that all the skills required can be combined in one person, the possibility of combining them within a health-care team seems realistic. It may be possible to use psychiatric nurses who have received training in interpersonal skills and counselling and who are also trained in general nursing. The high publicity given to the AIDS disease has proven to be of great interest to nurses, and it is reported that there is no shortage of nurses wishing to take up the challenge of nursing these patients.

The number of AIDS patients suffering with dementia or other psychiatric disorders does not yet seem to be large enough in the UK for the problem to have become a major concern for psychiatric nursing. However, AIDS patients are now beginning to present on inpatient psychiatric wards and outpatient departments, e.g. drug addiction clinics.

The divide which presently exists between psychiatric nurses and general nurses is acknowledged. It is suggested that there should be an interface between psychiatric nursing and general nursing, since AIDS patients need the skills of both groups, and an integrated service is required within which each group of nurses is able to assist the other. A possible solution to the problem is the use of liaison psychiatric nurses who could work on general wards with AIDS patients when required.

The problems highlighted by nurses also apply to other health-care workers, social services employees, prison officers and other personnel in contact with AIDS/HIV sufferers. On the one hand many of those working in areas where patients suffering from AIDS or AIDS-related conditions are cared for, have responded well to the demands that caring for people with this condition places upon them; on the other hand many remain prejudiced against client populations and/or phobic about contamination.

Some senior staff, for example, have negative attitudes and are prejudiced against AIDS sufferers. Sensationalist stories clearly demonstrate that, even with the present input of health education regarding AIDS, many health-care workers not only lack sufficient knowledge of the disease but also have a great deal of fear and misconception about it. This uninformed stance taken by some members within the health and social services highlights the need for continual education and updating of information about the condition. It is essential that information be continually disseminated to all those directly involved in providing care for persons with AIDS.

RESOURCE IMPLICATIONS

The lack of present resources, particularly in terms of manpower, must be stressed, especially for the future. There seems to be an ever-increasing gap between the rapid growth in need, with the number of AIDS sufferers steadily increasing, and the actual provision of adequate resources. The burden of coping with this lack of resources falls largely on those who are already involved in the care of AIDS patients. Inadequate staffing levels affect the health and safety of both the patients and the staff, which inevitably leads to low staff morale.

Present problems need to be clearly expressed and identified so that they may be solved. Health district general managers will require estimates of nursing staff and other resources to meet future needs. Careful co-ordination and planning between all disciplines is required in order to ensure the provision of a high-quality service.

IMPLICATIONS FOR TRAINING AND SUPERVISION OF AGENCY AND VOLUNTARY WORKERS

All training establishments have a considerable role to play in educating trainees on the subject of AIDS. All curricula should now include the subject in order to prepare health-care workers to face some of the issues raised in the management of this condition.

Continual education is probably the most effective method available to reduce prejudices against the minority groups presently affected: to reduce fear of contagion, and to portray an accurate and differential picture of AIDS and HIV-related conditions.

The importance of interpersonal skills and counselling skills has implications also for the training of health-care workers. While it is appreciated that certain disciplines, e.g. clinical psychologists and psychiatric nurses, have expertise in this field, it is stressed that all health-care workers should become skilled in these aspects of care, particularly since they play such an important part in the care of AIDS patients.

It is suggested that study days and courses on counselling should be available for all nurses, and although it is realised that there are a number of counselling courses available, the difficulty which remains, and which must be solved, is in arranging for staff to have the time to attend them.

AGENDA FOR RESEARCH

Two major areas of research are currently thought to require development.

Firstly research into the present attitudes of health care workers is required; the findings of this research would provide a baseline of the educational needs of these workers and direct appropriate educational programmes.

Secondly, information is required about the needs of AIDS patients as identified by themselves. In order to plan effective care for the future it seems necessary to monitor and evaluate the present care that these patients receive.

CONCLUSION

A diagnosis of AIDS has profound implications for the patient. The consequences are far-reaching for him/her, and may touch on every aspect of his/her life. More than any other condition AIDS has highlighted the need to see beyond the actual disease and to recognise the person and the psychosocial aspects of his/her life.

Caring for a patient with AIDS poses an immense challenge. This challenge can only be met by a concerted multidisciplinary effort. It is no longer a problem confined to venereologists, haematologists or immunologists, but is the concern of all.

The need for an integrated approach to the care of patients suffering with AIDS and related conditions is paramount. If safe, effective, and meaningful care to these patients is to be provided it is necessary for all available resources to be put to their best use.

By identifying the need for a conference to look specifically at the psychiatric and psychosocial aspects of AIDS and related conditions, and to provide a summary of the major issues involved, the first step has been taken in meeting this objective. The next step is the careful planning of detailed programmes to provide the care required. It is hoped that this chapter has highlighted some issues to be taken into account when planning such a programme.

5

Services for People Dependent on Drugs

J. Roy Robertson

This chapter is based on the discussions of a working group meeting specially convened for the purpose of considering services for people dependent on drugs who also develop AIDS. Professor J. Griffith Edwards, Professor of Addiction Behaviour, Institute of Psychiatry, London, was the chairman of the working group and the discussion was opened by Ms Jane Kennedy, AIDS Information Officer, Standing Committee on Drug Abuse (SCODA), London.

Dealing with people who are drug abusers, and who have AIDS, presents new difficulties for all health professionals who work in the field. The advent of AIDS on a drug-use scene, which is itself rapidly changing, has produced a widely varying pattern of problems throughout the country, which makes the introduction of new health-care services, and the modification of existing ones, an urgent requirement.

Since it is impossible in the short space available here to examine all areas of interest in this particular sphere, five main topics are considered in this chapter, which concludes with a statement of some aspects of the subject which are felt to be important and of urgent concern to those involved.

HIV INFECTION IN DRUG MISUSERS: THE SIZE OF THE PROBLEM

In Scotland 16 people have so far been confirmed as having AIDS, and of these 11 are dead. The number of seropositive tests recorded is 1,100 and of these 600–650 were drug users.

But the size of the problem is difficult to assess accurately, basically because the number of drug users cannot easily be estimated. In many areas such estimations are based on the Drug Indicators Project multiplication factor — i.e. five times the number of known drug users.

Whatever means are used to calculate the figures, however, it is important to have *some* basic information, such as the numbers of people using drugs, because such baseline data are essential if the effectiveness of therapy and treatment policies is to be appraised, and if proper resources for care and treatment are to be provided.

In this connection it is felt that local initiatives are most likely to produce the most accurate information; and the efforts are welcomed which the DHSS are making to modify collecting systems and more clearly to identify drugs which change injecting patterns — such as the increased use of amphetamines.

EDUCATION: ARE THE MASS MEDIA EFFECTIVE?

What is the real value of mass media programmes, the aim of which is to be educative in this field? Are they meant to be propaganda, or is their prime aim to provide information? Are they designed to effect change in the personal behaviour of individuals, or to give continuing support to sufferers?

The general view appears to be that the mass media could be effective in providing sufferers with continuing support, but is unlikely to be successful in changing patterns of behaviour. In an area of personal behaviour of enormous variation and complexity such intervention is superficial, and at best is only a first step in education.

There is manifestly a great need for information specifically aimed at high-risk activities. The difficulty is that networks

54

through which such information may effectively be disseminated do not seem to exist.

INTERVENTION

Professional staff who may be called upon to deal with people suffering from AIDS, especially in the sphere of drug misuse, badly need help and support in their work. How best may satisfactory educational arrangements be made?

Existing agencies with experience in drug misuse could well form the foundation of an appropriate professional educational substructure. Similarly experienced workers already in the drug field should be encouraged to have confidence in their own abilities to adapt and develop services.

Organisations which have the flexibility necessary for successful adaptation are more likely to be local than national, but there is a need for action nationally to encourage a spirit of collective responsibility, and to provide a means whereby information may be freely and usefully exchanged at both national and local levels.

FRONT LINE CARE: POLICY ISSUES

The advent of AIDS has served to focus attention on the treatment of drug abuse, and has helped to highlight problems which emerge from prescribing patterns, and from professional attitudes to treatment methods.

Debate will continue on the relative merits of drug misuser treatment based on non-prescribing, and that based on the prescription of alternatives such as methadone.

No-one would accept methadone prescribing as a panacea for all problems, but increasing its provision might offer a means of improving control over the spread of drug abuse and to some extent, of HIV.

There appear to be indications that current DHSS advice on methadone prescription may be undergoing some change.

NEUROPSYCHIATRIC MANIFESTATIONS OF AIDS

AIDS patients who are drug misusers and who become mentally disturbed as a result of their illness will need to be properly cared for. To this end appropriate management facilities must be made available, and adequate resources allocated for such provision.

Should this not be the case then the existing agencies and residential establishments will clearly be faced with serious problems.

Flexibility is important in providing new and appropriate management facilities, and the importance of testing for HIV antibody may need to be stressed.

It is essential that the impact of AIDS on the treatment of drug abuse be taken very seriously. Primary prevention and early treatment have now become much more important. In a complex and confusing situation there is, *inter alia*, a clear need for a multidisciplinary approach and for multidisciplinary fora where views, experience and advice may be shared.

FOOTNOTES

Finally it is worth drawing attention to some additional points relevant to the issue under consideration, but presented at random.

Drug users in prison for example, or those who are homeless, present special problems, as do the children of parents who are intravenous drug addicts.

Social factors such as unemployment and lack of proper housing can obviously exacerbate the problems, and point to the need for more action in the allocation of additional resources to, and a greater co-ordination of research in, this field of medical care and treatment. Action such as free needle exchange, and a greater emphasis on activities which can help to change drug using behaviour, would seem to be particularly worthwhile.

6

Young Children at Risk

Denise Platt

This chapter is based on the deliberations of a meeting of an interprofessional working group, chaired by Professor William Yule, Professor of Applied Child Psychology, Institute of Psychiatry, London, which came together to discuss the risks which young children run of contracting AIDS and AIDS-related conditions.

The meeting of the working group was opened by Professor Ivana Markova, Professor of Psychology at the University of Stirling, Scotland, and this chapter begins with an account of some of the issues which she raised.

WHO IS AT RISK?

Since the AIDS virus is transmitted by blood, and through sexual intercourse, potentially all children are at risk of AIDS if promiscuity continues to be a characteristic of the sex life of the younger generation. In addition, however, there are other groups of children who are at risk of becoming infected by the AIDS virus as passive recipients with no chance of taking any active steps against such danger. Two major groups of such children can be identified.

The first consists of children of drug-misusing parents who have been infected by the virus *in utero*. Evidence shows that, at present, seropositive drug-misusing women are still becoming pregnant and giving birth to children. Recently, six pregnancies of HIV-positive drug-misusing women were reported in Edinburgh, and two children, by now, have been born. Fortunately, they are both HIV-negative. However, there are at present about 300 drug-misusing women in Edinburgh who may eventually give birth to HIV-positive children.

The second group is made up of children receiving blood transfusions, and children who were infected by the virus through contaminated blood products, such as commercially produced factor VIII, and factor IX in the case of haemophilia A and B.

In the UK, by December 1986, 287 children were known to be in this group, but it should not increase in number because of the measures taken to screen blood donors and to heat-treat blood products. Indeed, the number of the youngest children, i.e. children under five years of age, who are infected by the HIV virus has considerably decreased since the above measures were taken.

In dealing with the problem of AIDS in children and adolescents it is therefore necessary to distinguish different tasks with which society must cope. If the view is accepted that, potentially, every child is at risk of acquiring the HIV virus, then the most effective programmes of sex education must be found. Those children who are already infected by the HIV virus require, in addition to effective sex education, a great deal of counselling and support in order to cope with their tragic situation. They may require hospitalisation and neurological treatment.

Bearing these problems in mind it seems that there are several issues that should be addressed.

INCIDENCE OF HIV POSITIVITY AND AIDS IN CHILDREN

Although AIDS is less common in children and adolescents than in adults, the number of children infected by HIV, and those suffering from AIDS-related conditions (ARC) and AIDS, is increasing.

In the USA, children with AIDS were first diagnosed in 1983. By July 1986, 321 children under 13 years with AIDS had been reported, of whom over 60 per cent had died. More than 75 per cent of these children acquired HIV infection *in utero*, or during birth, from their infected mothers. There is one report of a case from Sydney, Australia, which suggests that the child was infected through breast milk.

The number of children with AIDS in developing countries is not known, since there is no national reporting in those countries. Diagnosis is difficult because the symptoms of ARC and AIDS in children are non-specific, and are commonly expressed as a failure to thrive, diarrhoea, tiredness and loss of weight.

Statistics from the USA show that among children with AIDS, 60 per cent are black, 22 per cent Hispanic, and 18 per cent white. It is not known why there are such differences between the races. Are there genetic reasons for such differences? Does malnutrition in black and Hispanic children make them less resistant to the virus? If so, are children of drug misusers also at higher risk because they also are likely to suffer from malnutrition?

At Stirling, research into coping-strategies of people with haemophilia has demonstrated the particular problems of HIV-positive teenagers. Those in the 15–20-year age group usually either do not have a stable sexual relationship or have never had a sexual partner before.

Thus an angry young man recently said that 'all the birds he knew were on the pill' and he would feel 'a real charlie' if he produced a sheath. A more experienced patient, finding himself in a similar situation, had said to the girl that 'he was into rubber, it turned him on'.

The tragedy of the situation is that the individual drifts from one transient relationship to another. This enables him to cope without disclosing his status. Seeing a girl once or twice and drifting elsewhere frees him from the responsibility of telling her about his HIV positivity.

One of the major problems for those who are dependent on regular treatment by blood products, or on repeated blood transfusion, is to cope with double-messages concerning the safety of blood and blood products.

On the one hand it is claimed that these are safe, or at least that the likelihood of being contaminated by them is now extremely small. On the other hand, most Haemophilia Centres insist that everyone with haemophilia should be treated in the same way.

Thus the medical and nursing staff take the same kinds of precautions when treating haemophiliacs, whether they are HIV-positive or HIV-negative, and insist that everyone with haemophilia should take precautions with respect to their sex life and when treating themselves with factors VIII and IX.

How should teenagers with haemophilia and their parents interpret these double-messages?

It is very difficult for either to comprehend them, and this must inevitably cause distrust and worries among those concerned.

If there is a risk of contaminated blood and blood products this risk should be spelled out clearly, so that people can comprehend it and make decisions as to their behaviour accordingly. There is a good practice in genetic counselling of helping the counsellee to determine for himself or herself the acceptable level of risk with which he or she can live.

Effective sex education programmes will be required to make teenagers aware of the risk of contracting the AIDS virus and other sexually transmitted diseases. The trouble with many existing programmes is that they only provide young people with information about sex practices; it is more important that sex education programmes should make young people aware of the risk to them *as individuals*.

Thus a great deal of imagination and thought is required to develop education programmes directed towards the *individual* needs of young people. Such programmes will require highly skilled teachers, able to take the point of view of the young generation, and able to use language understood by the young. Both teaching and counselling skills are essential for everybody involved in sex education.

Turning now from the remarks of the opening discussant at the working group meeting, to the results of the general discussion, it is questioned whether the issue of AIDS in children is being treated seriously enough; whether it is seen as less pressing than the problems of adults; and whether the education system is being properly considered as an important vehicle of communication with young people.

THE IDENTIFICATION OF CHILDREN AT RISK

All children in today's society are at risk of becoming infected and catching AIDS, which makes this a major and urgent public health issue. It is felt that there are factors of high risk which can be identified for certain children, but that all children should be the target of any health education programme.

The factors of high risk are:

(1) haemophilia,

(2) affected mothers who put their unborn children at risk,

(3) sexually active adolescents;

(4) sexually abused children — a group who raise ethical issues concerning testing and screening,

(5) children beginning to experiment with drugs and exchanging needles, and

(6) young single homeless people who may turn to prostitution for money.

MEDICAL AND NURSING PROCEDURES

No particular medical procedures are necessary to deal with young children at risk, or who already have AIDS or the virus. It is important not to segregate such children from others, and simple hygienic precautions are all that is necessary to protect medical and nursing staff.

SPECIAL PROBLEMS IN WORKING WITH PARENTS, RESIDENTIAL ESTABLISHMENTS, FOSTER PARENTS AND ADOPTIVE PARENTS

A major issue is that of confidentiality, in particular confidentiality between agencies, and knowledge of how different agencies keep the information about people with AIDS on record.

In particular, the attitudes of some professionals who refuse to deal with people with AIDS — including children — could be an important factor in failing to pass on appropriate information.

There are also legislative dilemmas for local authorities which, for a number of children, stand *in loco parentis*. For example, for children in care who are infected, does the local authority tell the parents of other children in care placed in the same establishment or with the same foster parents?

How does the local authority deal with the dilemma of teenage girls (or boys for that matter) in care who, because they are promiscuous, may put other children in care at risk?

As for management issues concerning a child in a residential establishment, how will these issues be coped with within a social services department?

Should tests, for example, be undertaken automatically on children who have been sexually abused, and if so what about the issue of informed consent? What does informed consent *mean* in terms of a child who has been abused?

As already mentioned, regarding children with haemophilia who have contracted AIDS, their families are particularly angry at the message that AIDS is a sexually transmitted disease, because this somehow puts a 'slur' on their children's past behaviour.

One definition of confidentiality that has been proposed is that the information belongs to the parent and to the consultant, and only with the consent of the parent should the information be shared.

Regarding the implications of the Venereal Diseases Act, local authorities have responsibilities to all children in their care. In particular they must ensure that proper sex education is given to such children, and they are also responsible for educating all children about the issues, not only those who may be HIV-positive.

The management of the child who is known to be HIV-positive, however, should not be particularly different from that of other children in terms of life experience and growing up. It is acknowledged that talking to children and young people about sexual matters can create problems for staff, but largely these are training issues.

As for the emotional problems of staff in relation to AIDS, these are clearly important and must be addressed. It can be a strain on a professional if he or she is the only person outside the family to know that a child has AIDS. It is unfortunate that some families, sadly involved with a dying child, seem to be more preoccupied with a concern that the fact of the child having AIDS may be leaked outside the family, than with the important natural processes of bereavement and mourning that are so necessary for them emotionally.

CHILD'S SEXUAL KNOWLEDGE AND BEHAVIOUR

The important role of schools in the sex education of children is emphasised. The message to young people must be in a language which they can understand: current educational material and the AIDS campaign seem to be too formal to inspire serious attention in the young. The message should be about minimising risk, although it must be borne in mind that many young people do not see themselves as being at risk. It could well be that the most effective method of tackling this problem would be by means of small-group discussion of the issues involved.

Most young people's first sexual experience is unprotected, and many of them are undergoing an angry response — 'why us?'. The moral issues surrounding the debate are confusing to them. In adults, sex education and the AIDS educational programme is aimed at changing a behaviour that currently exists. In children and young people the aim is to influence a behaviour that has not yet been formed.

This can be quite problematic. What is proper sex education? How should it be given, and how explicit should it be? These are issues that have still to be faced.

Parents very often find it difficult to talk to their children about sexuality, and this can also be a problem for professionals involved with children — medical staff, teachers and social workers. Communication on sexuality is difficult for adults. Staff in residential establishments, hospitals, and similar institutions need to form a coherent view on the sex educational discussions which they intend to have with children.

Getting staff to agree a message on sexuality is not easy, and poses problems for adults who must sort out their own values and attitudes. How to make the necessary points in a language that is relevant to staff and children is a taxing issue.

The difficulties of sex education for children arise from the fact that the children need to see some result of action now, if they are to link current activities with future health.

Fortunately, however, there are positive experiences of changed sexual behaviour in young people; for example, in girls in relation to the pill and taking responsibility for their own sexual protection. This is a consequence of very rigorous sex education in schools and elsewhere.

Good publicity about the issues can also affect the behaviour of children. One example of this is the publicity given to child sexual abuse, which has resulted in a number of children approaching agencies for assistance. However, the essential effectiveness of a proper programme still needs to be addressed.

Recent government policy on sex education has devolved responsibility to individual schools, just at a time when it might be necessary to have a more comprehensive and overall programme. For example, some sex educational programmes can be unduly brief — half a day only — while others are quite extensive and spread over weeks. The new Special Health Education Authority may decide to make recommendations to the relevant government departments about the consequences of this new central policy.

RESOURCE IMPLICATIONS

It seems that the resource implications of AIDS can be described to use the old cliché, as yet another bottomless pit. However, specific implications are noted, specifically the lack of rehabilitation drug clinics in which mothers may be resident with their children. Clearly this is one important issue.

Another is that of educational programmes for staff at all levels and in all agencies — a need that it is impossible to quantify. Similarly no mention of financial allocations to local authorities in order to improve social work or domiciliary resources, has been made in recent government statements, which suggests that the important role of community care for people who have AIDS and who live at home is something that needs urgent attention.

IMPLICATIONS FOR TRAINING AND SUPERVISION OF AGENCY AND VOLUNTARY WORKERS

All professionals in all agencies need to understand the issue of AIDS, and the effects of dealing with people with AIDS in the context of their jobs. Training is particularly important for those in agencies who are the direct carers of people with AIDS. This involves not only nurses and doctors, but also home helps, foster parents, and day nursery staff.

All such workers must comprehend, from their various different professional and other viewpoints, how they are to address the issue of AIDS. Support for staff who come into contact with people with AIDS, and who worry about the problem, clearly needs to be provided.

These concerns can be manifested in either refusal to work with people with AIDS or in the creation of severe emotional problems in the staff involved. Support groups and discussion groups are very necessary in these circumstances. It should be noted, however, that while training is important in itself, so is the need to replace operational staff while they are on training courses.

This is no new problem, and discussions on AIDS and its implications merely highlight it, as they highlight other examples of past ineffectiveness in professional activities, such as in promoting good health and safety practices and in providing adequate bereavement counselling.

AGENDA FOR RESEARCH

What is needed is a comparative study of what activities and policies are effective in working with people with AIDS; an evaluation of different ideas, and a comparison in particular of different health education programmes. Some collation of the work currently being done is required so that it can be disseminated and good practices copied.

Information about normal sexual behaviour in young children is clearly important to those who are involved in working with this group and who seek to effect change in their attitudes. Equally important is research into what support networks are needed to assist families in the community when children have AIDS.

Finally, but most importantly, research into users' views of the service, and what they have found helpful about AIDS policies and procedures as these have affected them, is of key and paramount importance.

7

Social Problems, Emotional Symptoms and Psychiatric Disorders

John Green

This chapter is based on a discussion of the subject by a multiprofessional group at a special meeting chaired by Professor W.A. Lishman, Professor of Neuropsychiatry at the Institute of Psychiatry, London, and which had Dr T.W. Fenton, Consultant Psychiatrist at Hollymoor Hospital, Birmingham, to present the opening address.

The first part of the chapter consists of views put forward for consideration by Dr Fenton, and the second part reflects the main topics raised at the meeting by his fellow-members.

Dr Fenton points out that the social and emotional problems associated with HIV infection, and some of the psychiatric disorders also, are a reflection of the social stigma which has been attached to the disease, and which arises from intense anxiety about its contagious aspect. They reflect also the uncertainty surrounding HIV-positive status, and the usually fatal outcome of AIDS itself.

The fear that AIDS has so universally evoked in society is easily understood, and can be attributed to several well-established characteristics of the disease.

Since it was first identified the disease has spread in a virtually exponential way. There is every reason to believe that those infected, which of course includes the many who are seropositive but symptomless, will remain infectious thereafter, and may infect others without being aware that they are doing so.

Those who are seropositive but have not developed AIDS or ARC face a very uncertain and frightening future. They are aware that many of their number will succumb to AIDS, and they hear with anxious foreboding the gloomy speculations that most if not all will ultimately do so.

AIDS has been the subject of immense and often distorted, indeed seriously misleading, publicity. Wild and frightening accounts by the media have undoubtedly fanned the public hysteria surrounding AIDS and have encouraged prejudice against sufferers, their families and friends, and the social groups to which they may belong. Prejudice and discrimination have been exacerbated by identification of many of those infected to date with stigmatised minority groups, undermining the precarious tolerance which society had accorded those groups during one or two decades preceding the advent of the virus.

The irrational fears and negative discriminatory responses of the public, and tragically those of some health-care workers also, present constant problems to patients, their families and those concerned with their care.

There are many other stresses and pressures which arise from the progressive disablement and debilitation resulting from AIDS, and the growing dependency upon others; from loss of social and occupational status, and loss of earning capacity; from abrupt revelations of a hitherto private sexual preference, or dependence upon drugs, and from recognition that the patient is engaged with a lifestyle incurring social disapproval.

Family, friends and lovers may be distressed by a conflict between their love of the patient and the humiliation and social embarrassment of being closely associated with him. Confusion about the risk of transmitting infection to others, and about precautions that have to be followed, adds yet further stress, as does the need to sacrifice rewarding behaviours and lifestyles.

Identification of HIV-positive status may cause intense emotional perturbation, leading to suicidal ideas and behaviour, especially if the sufferer has received no preparatory counselling. As has been said, the diagnosis of AIDS itself is a catastrophic trauma, and is followed by emotional symptoms resembling those encountered with other life-threatening illnesses. These include shock and numbness, denial of illness, guilt and self-reproach, fear perhaps rising to panic, intense anger, and sadness with a deep sense of loss and anticipatory grief.

Taking all of these stresses into account, and recognising the high incidence of neurological complications in AIDS, it is surely no surprise to find that psychiatric disorders are a common association. As Dr Dilley has pointed out, these include anxiety reactions with marked hypochondriacal self-concern, depressive mood disorder, obsessive–compulsive disorder, psychoses associated with organic brain disease, dementia and in particular the AIDS dementia complex due to HIV encephalitis, and delirious reactions.

These may take a strong colouring and content from the particular psychic distress and existential plight of the individual who knows himself, or believes himself, to be infected with HIV, but it is important to appreciate that the psychiatric disorders associated with HIV infection are essentially syndromes with which psychiatrists are well familiar in other clinical contexts.

All of these considerations form the subject matter of this chapter. What are the implications for the medical, social and voluntary services? What needs to be done to alleviate these manifold problems and the distress that they occasion? What are the problems that beset health-care workers as they confront their patients and clients, and what are the implications for staff education and training?

Finally, from our exploration of the issues concerned, are we able to generate proposals for constructive avenues of research?

Looking now at some of the implications of the points made by Dr Fenton, let us first consider the question of education — and not just the need to educate the general public, but also the need in many instances, to educate our own staff about the issues surrounding AIDS.

A lot of the detail is contained within specialist journals and is not readily accessible to many people who are going to come into contact with this problem.

I believe that one of the difficulties we have is that if people knew more about the virus and the way that it works — if they knew more basic science about it — many of their fears would disappear. They would have information which they could generalise to different settings. And perhaps that is one of the mistakes we are making — we are providing generalised rules, rather than general information.

Secondly, there is the matter of confidentiality — the extent to which information needs to be kept confidential, and how it can be kept confidential.

It is broadly felt that with good general clinical practices, and good general hygiene, only those people who genuinely need to know within a hospital in order to treat the patient, should actually be informed of someone's HIV status.

It is also noted that National Health Service employees are covered by the sexually transmitted disease regulations and by their own contracts, which enforce confidentiality upon them.

Then there is the vexed issue of informed consent for testing, and the extent to which certain patients are able to give such consent.

While it is accepted that there may be individuals who cannot give informed consent (and in such circumstances it is not possible to obtain it) the general view is that the majority of patients, perhaps far more than we imagine, are actually capable of understanding the issues and of giving informed consent. Although in the past we have not always told our patients what tests we are carrying out on them, that may now be considered to be due to bad practice rather than to either common sense or what the law says we ought to be doing.

In this connection it must be borne in mind that matters concerned with life insurances, mortgages, and difficulties in employment are great problems for those who find that they are antibody-positive.

On the question of the amount of resources allocated to AIDS there is a general feeling that few if any of those involved in trying to deal with the problems are receiving enough money to undertake the various services which they wish to carry out, and that the local authorities are particularly hard-done-by in this respect.

The need is obvious for all involved, including the voluntary organisations concerned, to work together more closely in order to achieve an integrated strategy — thus ensuring that full use is made of the resources which are available in terms of staff skills and abilities.

On the subject of neuropsychology and psychiatric symptomatology, our experience at St Mary's Hospital, London, has been very different from that which Dr Dilley has described earlier. While there are signs that minor degrees of cognitive impairment may not be uncommon, we do not see nearly as many cases of florid AIDS-related dementia as have been reported from the USA, and colleagues in Australia say that their experience is similar to ours.

We do see a lot of AIDS-related dementia — really imitation dementia — which is the result of infection with opportunist infections of the brain itself. But while we certainly do see HIV dementia as such, we have not found it to be anything like as common as in the USA.

Whether that will change in the future I don't know. At this juncture I believe it to be an unlikely diagnosis in this country for a man with pre-senile dementia, but it is an issue which we are currently researching.

Secondly, on psychiatric symptomatology, again we seem to have a difference. We have seen over 200 patients at St Mary's, but we have only admitted one into a psychiatric unit, and that admission was for only about ten days and had nothing to do with AIDS. Generally speaking, therefore, from my own experience, I am sceptical of the proposition that there will be large numbers of AIDS patients who will need admission to psychiatric units.

A survey by my colleague, Heather George, showed that 60 per cent of our AIDS patients demonstrated no discernible psychiatric symptomatology at all. The other 40 per cent exhibited in the main mild depression or mild anxiety. Indeed, of all the AIDS patients we have had, only 19 per cent received anxiolitic medication — and then only for a period of a few weeks — and only 14 per cent had anti-depressant medication.

So the picture that we are seeing at St Mary's is very different from that in the USA. I do not understand why this should be the case, but taking a straw poll of colleagues who are dealing with AIDS patients in this country it would seem that at present their practice matches our own. We have never had a case of psychosis in an AIDS patient, and we have never had a suicide.

My own inclination as a result is strongly in favour of keeping patients on general wards rather than in psychiatric units, largely

71

I believe because of the difficulties of the reactions of other psychiatric patients, which cannot always easily be controlled, when they are told — as they may be by colleague patients — that they have AIDS.

Finally, when considering research, CNS involvement is manifestly a key area which is being investigated. But there are two others which seem to me to need more research.

The first is the issue of what I might describe as 'the worried well'. At St Mary's we receive 400 patients a month at a clinic who are 'worried well' people wanting blood tests. And it is the 'worried well' people who most often try to commit suicide and who have major psychiatric problems.

The second is concerned with the way in which we deliver health care. Information and advice is badly needed on the sort of services we should be providing, and how best they can be provided.

8

Counselling in Relation to HIV

Riva Miller

This chapter is the result of a special working group meeting which discussed the subject under the chairmanship of Dr David Miller, Senior Clinical Psychologist, Departments of Genito-Urinary Medicine and Psychiatry, Middlesex Hospital, London.

Garry Webb, AIDS Counsellor at the Camberwell Health Authority in London, gave the opening address to the multi-professional working group, and Mr Webb's comments are presented in the first part of the chapter, while the remainder is based on the discussions which subsequently ensued.

In the field of AIDS counselling the core issues that have to be dealt with — the practical matters if you like — depend very much on the philosophical basis from which counsellors approach the work they do, and how well they can resolve any conflict which exists between the philosophy and the practical issues of care.

An area of particular concern is the overall move that seems to be taking place, away from the concept of informed consent being given by patients, clients or individuals prior to their being tested. Not only is there no informed consent given, but in fact pre-test counselling is often either inadequate or non-existent. And as those involved in the counselling of people with AIDS know from personal and very sad experience, adequate pre-test counselling forms for them the whole foundation of the work that they can subsequently do, providing the parameters within which they can have any measure of success in dealing with the patients.

This particular trend away from pre-test counselling has implications for the rights of individual patients, and can affect their short-, medium- and long-term prognosis. It naturally affects the objectives of AIDS counselling, and can have important implications for the mental and emotional states of the patients, and so for the psychosocial support mechanisms they will require.

Manifestly, it has a further and basic effect — on resources — in terms of the number of people you need, the training they require, and their workload. It is unfortunate that the lead against pre-test counselling and informed consent seems to be coming from certain sectors of the medical profession and, from a counsellor's viewpoint, there would seem to be little or no identifiable good reason for this.

Counsellors would like to see the good working guideline followed, which is set out in the various departmental blue books and which is certainly accepted policy in some health regions, i.e. that people should have the test only after giving their informed consent, and after having had adequate pre-test counselling. And this latter proviso — what actually constitutes adequate pre-test counselling — is a key issue that has to be decided.

These are important matters if the role of counselling of this group of patients within the National Health Service is to be established, as opposed to leaving such counselling to voluntary organisations. That the interests of the client groups concerned be protected, is of over-riding importance.

In summary, then, this issue of pre-test counselling seems to parallel the way in which we in the health care field in the UK rehearse our response to the entire issue of AIDS in its broadest sense. Firstly it brings up the dilemmas of ethics, and the dilemma of whose prime interests our policy formation should basically represent. Should it be largely representative of those in the professional arena, or should it aim to serve the greater social good? Secondly, it also reflects the dilemmas of resource provision and training.

Turning, however, to the test itself, the reasons for wishing to have it will vary. We are, it could be said, a test-ridden society and some will favour the test as a safeguard for staff — managerial and other — as well as providing a means of deciding who has and who has not got HIV infection, and so helping us to understand the problem more. Human rights, however, may be very low on the list of priorities when tests are suggested.

An important point to be remembered in this general connection is that it is dangerous to separate test-counselling and testing from clinical settings. Perhaps an ethical group needs to be established to decide about this in all settings.

As for the objectives of counselling, there should be correct and consistent information about health education which should be so imparted that it is unbiased and helps people to make decisions that affect their behaviour.

Counselling should also relate to risk activity and not really to risk groups, and those undertaking what is called 'AIDS counselling', should of course themselves possess a very thorough knowledge of the subject.

On the question of what constitutes counselling, views vary, but basically it is considered to be the provision of ongoing support to individuals and their families. In addition, educating the public, providing training and support for staff and the giving of supervision, are additional aspects that must be taken into account. And of course it is important that counsellors counsel the patients rather than counsel about the disease.

Where is counselling to happen? Obviously it will take place in medical and in other settings, and in both it will need to be accompanied by appropriate training. Such training, education and counselling should start in the community and with youngsters, but there is also a need for education of medical and all other staff.

It is unsatisfactory that many patients who have been counselled in the large hospitals have then been referred on to voluntary agencies. This is seen as trying to obtain counselling 'on the cheap' because these agencies may well not have the resources to undertake the tasks forced upon them.

In order to help in this respect, and to match more closely the available resources to the demands of the client group, it seems appropriate to consider group counselling, as an alternative —

temporarily — to the appointment of more counsellors, so obviously needed.

At the present time, because knowledge of AIDS and HIV infection is very complicated, even for professionals, it would seem sensible to arrange for counselling to be undertaken by specially trained staff working in special centres with specialist facilities.

Several other areas of concern exist in the sphere of AIDS counselling, one being the stigma which attaches to the client group and so to the counsellors themselves.

It is a worrying thought for the future that many AIDS counsellors — designated AIDS counsellors — are not on long-term contracts, and of equal concern is the workload they may be asked to bear.

One suggestion is that counsellors should be limited to a given number of clinical hours a week — say 18 — with the warning that if they do more than that they are entering into a danger zone.

Another is that AIDS counsellors should work full-time but only spend a specified part of their time dealing directly with patients. It is recognised that actually changing jobs on a part-time basis could prove to be difficult in practice.

In this connection it is also suggested that client groups themselves could become their own support and counsellors, as has happened already with groups such as Body Positive. Counsellors should certainly not be expected to devote the whole of every working week to AIDS; they should do something else for some part of the time.

Finally it is important to emphasise the need for very close liaison between counsellors and other appropriate professionals, so that clients who receive counselling do not return to the care of other health-care staff ignorant of the form and objectives of the counselling.

Everyone is now well aware of the psychosocial input necessary to the proper care and treatment of people suffering from AIDS and other illnesses and diseases which can only be appropriately tackled on a multidisciplinary basis.

9

Epilogue

J.L. Reed

The conference on the 'Psychiatric and Psychosocial Aspects of AIDS and Related Conditions', held at the Institute of Psychiatry, London 27 February 1987, upon which this book is based, was a uniquely stimulating and informative occasion attended by representatives of an unusually wide variety of agencies.

Staff of voluntary organisations, probation officers, social workers, nurses working in hospitals, in the community and industry, doctors — both specialists in psychiatry and other clinical areas, and general practitioners, psychologists, counsellors, and many more, met together to discuss the major public health issue of our time.

The meeting marked a major step forward in our understanding of the psychiatric and psychosocial aspects of HIV infection and AIDS, and from its deliberations and discussions five topics emerged which merit the serious consideration of everyone involved in the battle against AIDS and related conditions.

Firstly there is a great need for more and better information on HIV infection and AIDS. The conference identified not only the need for more research information about the psychiatric symptomatology of HIV infection and its natural history, but also the need for wider information for the general public. It was suggested during the conference that the biggest single problem is the public's 'phobia' of AIDS. Only education will overcome unreasoning fear and replace it with the reasoned caution that is necessary to control the spread of HIV infection.

The second topic was related to the first, and addressed the need for training for those who will be involved in the care of AIDS sufferers with psychiatric symptoms. How far are additional skills, as opposed to special knowledge, needed to cope with the problems of the psychiatric symptoms of AIDS and related conditions?

The third topic related to ethical problems. These stretch far beyond the medical ethical problems relating to, for instance, HIV testing, whether of individuals or of groups. AIDS presents all of us, whether as professionals or as members of the general public, with new and as yet unresolved ethical dilemmas.

Related to ethical problems is the fourth topic — that of confidentiality. The problem of what information should be passed between specialist medical services and general practitioners was raised on several occasions, as was the responsibility of the general practitioner to those partners of HIV-positive patients who might also be his patients. The conference made it clear that problems of confidentiality of information, concern all who are involved with people who are HIV-positive, and questioned to what extent the present understanding of confidentiality adequately covers the new situation.

The final topic raised was that of priorities, with questions as to how the needs of AIDS sufferers should fit in with existing national priorities.

HIV infection presents us with a new range of problems, many of which will need further consideration and research so that we can move forward in the most appropriate way. The conference has had a very important function not only in disseminating knowledge but also in helping to define an agenda for further discussion.

There are, however, areas where we have a clear indication of future need. We know, for instance, that established cases of AIDS will spend a minority of their time in hospital, and that the major part of care will be in the community. This re-emphasises the need for health and social services to plan together and to work closely with housing departments and the voluntary sector in order to produce the wide range of services that will be required to meet the needs of AIDS sufferers.

In conclusion it is important to mention some of the action already under way relating to the psychiatric aspects of HIV infection. The Expert Advisory Group on AIDS (EAGA) has a psychiatric sub-group whose remit is 'to consider the diagnostic problems of psychiatric disease in AIDS patients, its likely prevalence, its management problems and to produce relevant guidance'. A report of the conference will be considered by the sub-group.

In order to promote effective national action in combating the spread of AIDS all health districts have been asked to develop plans of action concentrating on high-risk groups, complementing the national publicity campaign and including provision for testing, counselling services and for treating clinical cases of AIDS. Many districts have now completed this task, and the results are being considered.

A working group has been established by the Department of Health and Social Security to draw up guidelines for policy and practice in relation to AIDS for personal social services.

Following discussions with the Home Office a new drug misuse notification form, which will yield improved information on injecting behaviour, is being introduced in July/August 1987. This will materially contribute to our ability to target services for AIDS.

There are two important additional ways in which doctors can help improve information about AIDS.

Firstly there is the PHLS Communicable Diseases Surveillance Centre's national surveillance scheme for AIDS. This is based on voluntary confidential reports from clinicians. Full reporting is most important and CDSC would be happy to discuss the scheme with any doctors who are uncertain about it.

Secondly, information on a high-risk group can be improved by more complete notification of drug-misusers. Those patients who misuse drugs and who should be notified to the Chief Medical Officer often go unreported. Doctors, who have a statutory duty to notify should be sure to complete and return the notification forms.

Large though the number of people were who attended, or wanted to attend, the conference at the Institute of Psychiatry, it is likely that even more people will be needed to declare an interest in working on the problems presented by AIDS. It is incumbent on us all to persuade colleagues to take a personal interest in this vital problem.

Appendix 1

LIST OF GUIDANCE ISSUED BY THE DHSS AND OTHER GOVERNMENT DEPARTMENTS (APRIL 1987)

AIDS Some Questions and Answers. (DES)
Facts for Teachers, Lecturers and Youth Workers. Available from: the Publications Despatch Centre, DES, Honeypot Lane, Stanmore, Middlesex. February 1987.

Protect your Health Abroad. (DHSS)
Advice to travellers about the dangers of AIDS overseas. Leaflet SA 35 1987. Available from DHSS Leaflets Unit, Honeypot Lane, Stanmore, Middlesex HA7 1AY. November 1986 Print.

Acquired Immune Deficiency Syndrome (AIDS). DHSS
General information for doctors by expert advisory group on AIDS. Available from DHSS Publications Unit, Heywood, (Lancs). May 1985.

Possible infection risk to laboratory staff from human blood-based coagulation factor-deficient plasmas. DHSS
Available from DHSS Store, Health Publications Unit, No. 2 Site, Manchester Road, Heywood, Lancs OL10 2PZ. 1985. Safety information bulletin SIB (85) 30.

HTLV III infection in laboratory workers. DHSS
Available from DHSS Medical Branch, Alexander Fleming House, Elephant and Castle, London, SE1 6BY. DCMO (85) 2. December 1985.

Information for doctors concerning the introduction of the HTLV III antibody test. DHSS
Available from DHSS Store, Health Publications Unit, No. 2 Site, Manchester Road, Heywood, Lancs OL10 2PZ. OMO (85) 12. 1985.

Acquired immune deficiency syndrome (AIDS): HTLV III antibody testing outside the national blood transfusion service (NBTS)
Available from DHSS Store, Health Publications Unit, No. 2 Site, Manchester Road, Heywood, Lancs OL10 2PZ. OMO (85) 11. 1986 Reprint.

HTLV III antibody testing of blood donations outside the National Blood Transfusion Service (NBTS)
Available from DHSS Health Services Division 1A, Hannibal House, Elephant and Castle, London SE1 6TE. DA (86) 1. 1986.

Public Health Laboratory Service and Department of Health and Social Security evaluation of ten commercial anti-HTLV III/LAV assay kits.
Available from DHSS STD3, room 320, 14 Russell Square, WC1B 5EP. STB (86) 14. 1986.

Advisory Committee on Dangerous Pathogens LAV/HTLV III: the causative agent of AIDS and related conditions: revised guidelines.
Available from DHSS Health Publications Unit, No. 2 Site, Manchester Road, Heywood, Lancs. OL10 2PZ. HN (86) 20. 1986.

AIDS and artificial insemination: guidance for doctors and AI clinics: Acquired immune deficiency syndrome Booklet 4.
Available from DHSS Health Publications Unit, No. 2 Site, Manchester Road, Heywood, Lancs OL10 2PZ. CMO (86) 12. 1986.

Children at school and problems related to AIDS. DHSS
Available from DHSS Store Health Publications Unit, No 2 Site, Manchester Road, Heywood, Lancs OL10 2PZ. CMO (86) 10. 1986.

Children at school and problems related to AIDS. DES and Welsh Office. 1986.
Available from Publications Despatch Centre, Canons Park, Middx, HA7 1AY. (DES) Information Division, Cathays Park, Cardiff, CF1 3NQ. (Welsh Office).

AIDS: guidance for surgeons, anaesthetists, dentists, and their teams in dealing with patients infected with HTLV III. Booklet 3. DHSS
Available from DHSS Health Publications Unit, No 2 Site, Manchester Road, Heywood, Lancs, OL10 2PZ. CMO (86) 7. CNO (86)7. 1986.

AIDS: guidance for local authority staff.
Available from DHSS Store, Health Publications Unit, No. 2 Site, Manchester Road, Heywood, Lancs OL10 2PZ. LASSL (86) 8. 1986.

Public Health Laboratory Service and DHSS evaluation of Ortho Diagnostics, HTLV III Elisa Test.
Available from DHSS STD3, Room 320, Russell Square, London WC1B 5EP. STD (86) 38. 1986.

Microbiology Advisory Committee. Decontamination of equipment, linen, or other surfaces contaminated with hepatitis B or HIV.
Available from DHSS Store, Health Publications Unit, No. 2 Site, Manchester Road, Heywood, Lancs OL10 2PZ. Enclosure to HN (87) 1. 1987.

AIDS and employment. DOE
Available from AIDS and Employment, The Mailing House, Leeland Road, London W13 9HL. No Reference. 1986.

AIDS: What you must know before you give blood. NBTS
Information for blood donors only. Available from Information Division, Rm D51276, Alexander Fleming House, London SE1 6BY. NBTS. 1181 Sept. 86.

Appendix 2: AIDS/HIV Support Groups

There follows a list of support groups dedicated to persons with AIDS or HIV infection. As new groups are frequently being formed, the list is by no means exhaustive, and if a group is not listed for your area or region, check with your local genito-urinary medicine clinic (STD), which may have knowledge of local groups.

East Anglia Region
Cambridge AIDS Help Group,
287 Newmarket Road,
Cambridge CB5 8JE.

Mersey Region
Merseyside AIDS Support Group,
63 Shamrock Road, Birkenhead,
Merseyside L41 0EG.
Telephone line: 051 7080234. Wed 7–10 pm.

Northern Region
AIDS North,
PO Box 1BD,
Newcastle Upon Tyne NE99 1BB.

Northern Ireland
Cara-friend,
PO Box 44,
Belfast BT1 1SH.
Telephone lines: Belfast 222023. Mon–Thurs 7.30–10.00 pm.
Londonderry 263120. Thurs 7.30–10.00 pm.

North Western Region
Manchester AIDS Line,
PO Box 201,
Manchester M60 1PU.
Telephone line: 061 2281617. Mon, Wed, Fri 7–10 pm.

Oxford Region
OXAIDS, c/o Harrison Department,
Radcliffe Infirmary,
Oxford.
Telephone line: 0865 246036. Wed 6–8 pm.

Oxford Body Positive,
Freepost, Nether Westcote,
Oxford OX7 6BR.
Telephone line: 0865 246036.

Reading Area AIDS Support Group,
PO Box 75, Reading,
Berkshire.
Telephone line: 0734 503377. Thurs 8–10 pm.

Milton Keynes AIDS Support Group,
PO Box 153, Wolverton,
Milton Keynes.
Telephone line: 0908 312196. Mon 7–9 pm.

Scotland
Scottish AIDS Monitor,
PO Box 169,
Edinburgh, Scotland.
Telephone line: 031 5581167. Tues 7–10 pm (ansaphone at other times).

AIDS Information and Counselling Service,
129 Kilmarnock Road,
Shawlands, Glasgow G41 3YT.

South Western Region,
Aled Richards Trust,
1 Mark Lane,
Bristol BS1 4XR
Telephone: 0272 297963
Helpline: 0272 273436 (Mon–Fri 7–9 pm)

Thames Regions
North East Thames
Camden AIDS,
Area Three Social Services,
West End Lane, London NW6

PASAC, PO Box 130,
Colchester, Essex.
Telephone line: 0206 560225. Mon, Wed 7–9 pm

North West Thames
Bedford Gay Helpline,
38 Cherry Walk, Kempston,
Bedford.

South East Thames
Medway and Maidstone Gay Switchboard,
PO Box 10C,
Chatham, Kent ME4 6TX.
Telephone line: 0634 826925. Thurs/Fri 7.30–9 pm.

Sussex AIDS Helpline,
PO Box 17, Brighton BN2 5NQ.
Telephone line: 0273 734316. Mon–Fri 8–10 pm.

South West Thames
CALM, PO Box 11,
Bognor Regis, West Sussex PO21 1AH.
Telephone line: 0243 776998. Mon, Wed, Fri 7–9.30 pm

Trent Region
Nottingham AIDS Info Group,
Sharespace, 49 Stoney Street,
Nottingham.
Telephone line: 0602 585526. Mon, Tues 7–10 pm.

Wessex Region
Bournemouth AIDS Support Group,
PO Box 263,
Bournemouth BH8 8DY.
Telephone line: 0202 38850. Mon, Tues 8–10 pm.

Solent AIDS Line,
PO Box 139,
Southampton, Hants.
Telephone line: 0703 37363. Tues, Thurs, Sat 7.30–10 pm.

West Midlands
AIDS Concern Midlands,
79 Stanmore Road,
Edgbaston, Birmingham B16 9SU.
Telephone line: 021 6221511. Tues 7.30–9.30 pm.

Yorkshire Region
Bradford Gay Switchboard Collective,
643 Littlehalton lane,
Bradford BD5 8BY.
Telephone line: 0274 42895. Sun, Tues, Thurs 7–9 pm.

Leeds AIDS Information and Counselling Service,
11 Plaintree View,
Shadwell, Leeds 17.

Leeds AIDS Line,
64–68 Call Lane,
Leeds LS2.
Telephone line: 0532 441661. Tues 7–9 pm.

West Yorkshire AIDS Support Group,
1 Cambridge Street,
Hebdon Bridge, West Yorkshire HX7 6LN.

Irish Republic
Gay Health Action,
10 Fownes Street,
Dublin 2, Eire.
Telephone line: Dublin 710939. Mon–Fri 11 am–4 pm.

National Groups
The Terrence Higgins Trust,
BM AIDS,
London WC1N 3XX.

The Terrence Higgins Trust is a registered charity which offers help and advice to AIDS sufferers and their significant others. In addition, they offer a 'buddy volunteer' scheme, for people living in London, aimed at befriending and helping those with AIDS. Telephone number: 01-278 8745.

Body Positive,
BM AIDS,
London WC1N 3XX.

Body Positive is a national support and advisory group for those infected with the HIV virus. It is entirely voluntary, and operates from a base in London.

The Haemophilia Society,
PO Box 9, 16 Trinity Street,
London SE1 1DE.
Telephone number: 01-407 1010.

The Haemophilia Society offers help, advice and support to those persons suffering from haemophilia, and their families.

Standing Conference on Drug Abuse (SCODA) Ltd,
1–4 Hatton Place, Hatton Garden,
London EC1N 8ND.
Telephone number: 01-430 2341.

SCODA co-ordinates activities of non-statutory agencies in the drug field. It also publishes detailed guides to specialist drug services throughout the country.

The Nurses Support Group,
53 Mirlees Court, Camberwell,
London SE5 9QW.
Telephone number: 01-274 5442.

The Nurses Support Group offers advice and help to health care providers with HIV problems.

London Lighthouse,
178 Lancaster Road,
London W11 1QU.

London Lighthouse is a charitable project to establish a hospice incorporating a small residential unit to act as a continuing care facility for those persons with AIDS. In time, it will provide a counselling, training and information service.

Organisations giving advice to the public on AIDS.

(1) Terrence Higgins Trust
    BM/AIDS London WC1N 3XX
    Telephone Helpline (01) 833 2971
    Mon–Fri 7–10 pm
    Sat–Sun 3–10 pm

(2) Healthline Telephone Service
    01-981 2717, 01-980 7222, 0345 581151
    For recorded information on AIDS 24-hour service. For calls from outside London, the 0345 number will be charged at local rates

(3) London Lesbian and Gay Switchboard
    01-837 7324

(4) SCODA (Standing Conference on Drug Abuse)
    1–4 Hatton Place, London EC1N 8ND
    01-430 2341

(5) The Haemophiliac Society
    PO Box 9, 16 Trinity Street, London SE1 1DE
    01-407 1010
    Advice for haemophiliacs and their partners

Index

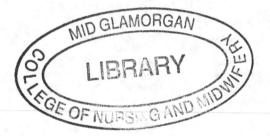